# Praise for
# *The Doula Advantage*

"If you're expecting a baby, you owe it to yourself to read this book! With a friendly tone and practical examples, Rachel Gurevich explains what doulas are, what they do, and how these special caregivers can help you have a better birth. With words of wisdom from perinatal, birth, and postpartum doulas—together with feedback from the moms they have helped—*The Doula Advantage* is a must for any pregnant woman."

> —NANCY PRICE
> Editor-in-Chief, ePregnancy.com
> and *ePregnancy* magazine

"This book shows the powerful and beneficial role of the doula in today's maternity care scene. It contains a wealth of information and practical suggestions that can be used while hiring and employing the services of a doula."

> —PAULINA G. (POLLY) PEREZ, BSN, FACCE, CD
> Author of *Special Women: The Role of the Professional Labor Assistant* and *Doula Programs: How to Start and Run a Private or Hospital-Based Program with Success*

"As a childbirth professional since 1989, I would highly recommend *The Doula Advantage* to anyone considering using a doula or becoming one. The book is well written, easy to read, and includes an excellent list of resources for doulas and families."

> —TRACY WILSON PETERS, ICCE, CLD, CLE
> CAPPA Founder and Executive Director
> www.cappa.net

"*The Doula Advantage* is a must-read for any woman thinking of using the services of a doula. The book is comprehensive, thought-provoking, and highly moving. Rachel Gurevich does an outstanding job of making the case for doula care and paying tribute to the very important work that doulas do on behalf of laboring women."

> —ANN DOUGLAS, author of *The Mother of All Pregnancy Books* and *The Mother of All Baby Books*

# The Doula Advantage

*Your Complete Guide to Having an Empowered and Positive Birth with the Help of a Professional Childbirth Assistant*

*Rachel Gurevich*

PRIMA PUBLISHING

Copyright © 2003 by Prima Publishing, a division of Random House, Inc.

Published by Prima Publishing, Roseville, California. Member of the Crown Publishing Group, a division of Random House, Inc.

PRIMA PUBLISHING and colophon are trademarks of Random House, Inc., registered with the United States Patent and Trademark Office.

**Library of Congress Cataloging-in-Publication Data**
Gurevich, Rachel.
    The doula advantage : your complete guide to having an empowered and
    positive birth with the help of a professional childbirth assistant / author,
    Rachel Gurevich.— 1st ed.
        p. ; cm.
    Includes bibliographical references and index.
    ISBN 0-7615-0058-8
    1. Doulas. [DNLM: 1. Allied Health Personnel. 2. Labor. 3. Midwifery.
WQ 300 G979d 2003] I. Title.
RG950 .G875 2003
618.4'5—dc21                                                      2002155156
                                                                        Rev.
03 04 05 06 HH 10 9 8 7 6 5 4 3 2 1
Printed in the United States of America
First Edition

**Visit us online at www.primapublishing.com**

*To my husband and very best friend, Eliyahu.*
*May we share many happy years together.*

*And to my children, Menachem and Eliezer.*
*May you both be blessed with health and happiness.*

# Contents

## Part One:
## Introduction to the Doula

## Part Two:
## The Labor Doula

# Part Three:
# The Postpartum Doula

# Part Four:
# The Antepartum Doula

# Part Five:
# Becoming a Doula

# Foreword

THE *DOULA ADVANTAGE* exquisitely outlines the role of the doula in labor, delivery, postpartum care, and breastfeeding and discusses how to hire a doula. Homefirst Health Services, the medical group I founded, has used doulas for more than 10 years.

The primary problem with American obstetrics is the inordinately high cesarean section rate, which is approaching 30 percent of all births. Cesarean section has a 5 to 10 times greater morbidity and mortality rate for both newborns and mothers than does vaginal delivery. America ranks between 24th and 26th in the world in infant and maternal mortality. If you look at the countries with the best rankings, you will also notice that they have the lowest percentage of cesarean sections.

As this book points out, the doula plays an integral part in the labor and delivery process, bringing emotional, physical, and practical support to the laboring woman. Medical studies have shown that women who require pain medication during labor will have a higher percentage of cesarean sections. Even though the doula does not play a direct medical role in the delivery and postpartum process, the comfort measures that she provides empower the woman to labor more effectively. This helps lessen the need for pain medication, and many times no pain medication is needed, thereby reducing the percentage of cesarean sections. I have always liked simple analogies that have profound effect. Michael Eisner, CEO of Disney, once stated, "Quality is when the reality exceeds the expectation." It has been my personal, as well as professional, experience that having doulas present at birth meet this definition of quality. The presence of a doula helps the reality of labor and birth exceed the laboring mother's expectation.

I highly recommend *The Doula Advantage* for women who are thinking about getting pregnant, are pregnant, or who have just given birth—as well as for anyone interested in how to become a doula. Kudos to Rachel Gurevich for bringing such an important topic to the public forum.

*—Mayer Eisenstein, M.D., J.D., M.P.H.*
*author of* The Home Birth Advantage

# Preface

I HAVE ALWAYS LOVED the feeling of being pregnant and thought of the entire process of pregnancy through birth to motherhood as an exciting journey. Of course, pregnancy and birth come with challenges. I'm the type of person who suffers from morning sickness from conception to birth! But this never stopped me from loving the concept of having a little person grow inside me.

When I first realized I was pregnant with my second son, I was thrilled. I decided to get into a *birthing mood* early and read some birth stories. As I started to read, and the woman in the story was describing her feelings during the first hours of labor, I began to feel sick. I needed to lie down and close my eyes, and asked my husband to bring me a cool cloth for my forehead. I didn't understand why, but my heart was pounding and a high-pitched ring stung in my ears. Something about the story made me ill, though I hadn't at the time understood why.

A few days later, I tried reading a different birth story. And again, I felt my heart pounding, lay down, and this time, I actually vomited. Then I started having nightmares: of being alone during birth, of giving birth to a deformed child. Why was this happening to me? What was so upsetting about reading a birth story, something I had loved to do during my first pregnancy?

After much introspection and conversation with a dear friend, I realized I was experiencing a sort of post-traumatic stress. As I will briefly describe in the first chapter of this book, my first birth was difficult emotionally. I had not realized how much the birth affected me until I was pregnant with my second son.

I had planned on hiring a doula for my second child's birth, but now I knew it was an absolute necessity for me. I began my search early and with each doula I spoke to, I related my first birth experience. Talking about the birth seemed to make me feel more at peace, and the doulas that I interviewed always listened and understood.

I read every book I could find on birth and childbirth methods. I studied books on Jewish meditation, for use during labor, and I prayed for an easy and calm birthing experience. I purchased Hypnobirthing tapes and listened to the affirmations tape daily. With light, bell-like music in the background, I would listen, "I turn my birthing over to my natural birthing instincts . . . My mind is relaxed. My body is relaxed. My birthing muscles work in complete harmony to make my birthing easier. I feel confident. I feel safe. I feel secure. I release, and I let go. . . ." This may sound corny to you, but it was extremely powerful for me. As I listened to the tapes over and over, I started to really believe what was being said.

My doula, Diane Lentine, provided the perfect support for me. I had a calm and beautiful birth. There were no interventions, and I was not frightened. I was so calm during the birth that my doctors commented they never saw anyone "sleep" through transition. We named our son, Eliezer, meaning *my God helped me,* in recognition of God's obvious mercy on me during the baby's birth.

Perhaps you are considering the idea of hiring a doula, but are hesitating. You may be wondering exactly what a doula can do for you that your family, partner, or friend cannot. You may be worried that a doula will push you into a certain way of birthing, or that the doula will not be worth the money. Or perhaps you're sure you want a doula, but you don't know where to begin your search . . . or how to pay.

I hope this book will answer your questions and reassure any doubts you have. I look back at my first birth experience, and I know a doula would have made a world of difference. I believe every woman deserves a doula, and I know many more women would seek support if they understood the role of the doula better and knew how to find and hire one.

In writing this book, I tried to be as inclusive as possible, without ruining the language or confusing my readers. I understand that there are many different types of families. I have used the words "husband" and "partner" interchangeably in the book, and I do know some women may be going through pregnancy and birth alone.

I use the term *normal birth* the same way many people use the term *natural* (or *nonmedicated*) *birth*. There is a great amount of dispute over what natural birth is. Is it *natural* to give birth in a hospital? Is a birth not *natural* if a fetal monitoring device is used? When I say normal birth, I simply mean a birth that does not need any additional help from medications, either pain relief, induction medication, or others; and does not involve the use of invasive procedures, such as forceps, episiotomy, or cesarean section.

I want to make clear that I am not judging those that choose medication, as I myself used medication in the birth of my first child. But medication is something added into the equation, and therefore is not the typical way your body would birth. Sometimes medication is necessary. I respect that, and so should any doula that you hire.

Please share this book with any pregnant friend, even if they assure you that a doula is not for them. There are many misconceptions about doulas, and by sharing this book with others, you are helping to educate the world on how doulas can help women have more positive birth and postpartum experiences.

PART ONE

# Introduction
# to the Doula

# Who Are These Special Women?

W<small>HEN</small> I <small>WAS EXPECTING</small> my first child, I received unsolicited advice from everyone—from the cashier at the pharmacy ("Are you sure you want to buy that pregnancy test?") to older women who happened to walk by me on the street ("Make sure you eat more fiber! Prunes will do you good for that constipation!"). There were those close to me who offered good advice. But I often ignored it, being naïve and overwhelmed by the barrage of comments from strangers.

"Will someone be with you in the labor room?" Sara, a mother who had given birth several times previously, asked me.

"My husband will," I answered. "We took a class." Sara looked up from her cleaning in the kitchen.

"Rachel, he's not going to be able to help you as much as you need. Will someone be there who is experienced with birth? Another woman?"

"My best friend will be there," I said. "I think it will be all right."

My best friend, though she had zero experience with childbirth and pregnancy, was ready to hold my hand and help support me. I assumed my husband would remember the techniques we learned in childbirth education class. Personally, I read as many books on childbirth as I could. I thought I was ready. I thought it would be okay.

But it didn't turn out *okay*.

Much of the information I remembered from birth books and childbirth class I used incorrectly, partially because I was nervous and excited, partially because this was my first time. I remembered reading that a woman should not eat or drink during childbirth, but I didn't realize they meant true labor—not prelabor.

I arrived at the hospital too early. The doctor decided to break my water to "get things moving," something I wished they hadn't done, but didn't know I could refuse. My husband tried to coach me in breathing exercises, but he thought hyperventilating was the correct way and slow breathing was incorrect.

My friend did exactly what I expected. She held my hand. But she also looked at me like she was sure I would die, which didn't help my confidence. My mother was there, but she was overwhelmed watching her daughter give birth and not in the position to support or coach me.

I found the hospital environment intimidating. The nurses walked in and out of the room without even saying hello to me. I don't think I was once told their names. They positioned me on my back to strap on the fetal monitors, and a few minutes later I started to pass out. Lying on your back for extended periods of time in late pregnancy is dangerous because the weight of the uterus pushes on vital blood vessels. I called for a nurse to help me, and she had me lie on my side. I felt so helpless that I didn't even think to reposition myself until someone told me I was "permitted" to move.

I asked for some water but was only allowed ice chips. Because I'd had no fluids the entire day, I was feeling ill and needed hydration. After a couple of hours, my husband asked a nurse when they would check my cervical dilation.

"Whenever she asks for drugs," the nurse replied.

My husband, knowing I wanted to give birth normally, asked, "What if she never asks for drugs?"

"Oh, she will!" the nurse laughed. "I wouldn't have given birth to three children if it weren't for the drugs!" This happened in 1999, and from my work with doulas and women, things have not changed—and this attitude is common in all different parts of the country.

At that point, I felt no hope. I was exhausted, thirsty, and lonely. I didn't know it, but I was going through transition. I asked for an epidural and was told it would be another hour before the anesthesiologist could administer the medication. Ironically, my first experience with a doula came when I was given the epidural.

It is extremely important to stay still when an epidural is administered. I was scared to death. I knew I would have at least one or two contractions while they inserted the epidural catheter.

"We will work through them, and you will be okay," the nursing assistant assured me. Touching my arm, she looked straight into my eyes and said softly, "Breathe normally, in and then out . . . that's it, relax."

I sat up in the bed, resting my head on her shoulder while the anesthesiologist administered the epidural. When I started having a contraction, I began to panic. The nursing assistant's voice and words calmed me, more than I would have expected.

"Take a deep breath, Rachel. And now, breathe out, try to relax your muscles, let the contraction happen . . . breathe in . . . and breathe out . . . don't fight your body, just let it happen. They peak, and then they fade away . . . it's almost over, take a nice, cleansing breath . . . very good."

The two contractions that she coached me through were magical. The pain wasn't unbearable anymore. I felt more in control. As they helped me lie back down on the bed, I felt intense pressure. They examined me, and it was time to push the baby out. One hour later, my baby was born.

If only I had had the emotional and physical support of a doula the entire time, I know I could have birthed normally. I made a mental promise not to labor without an experienced labor coach for my next child. I did hire a doula for my second baby's birth, and I did give birth normally with no interventions. I actually enjoyed labor and never felt out of control or helpless. I still felt pain, but my anxiety and fears were lessened. It was truly a wonderful experience.

# What Is a Doula?

A doula is a professional who provides emotional, physical, informational, and practical support for the expectant, laboring, or postpartum mother. She does not perform any medical tasks but actually complements the medical birth team. The word *doula,* pronounced /doo-la/, comes from the Greek and is loosely translated as "woman servant." Usually when people use the word, they are referring to a labor doula, but there are two other kinds: postpartum and antepartum doulas. While some provide both labor and postpartum services, the majority specialize in one of the three areas.

### ANTEPARTUM DOULA

An antepartum doula provides emotional and practical support for pregnant women. She may help the mother-to-be by doing light

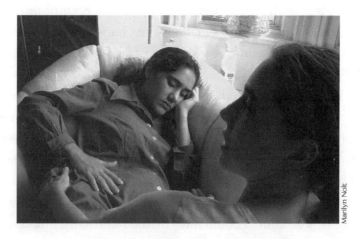

FIGURE 1.1. With her doula's support,
this mother is able to relax and labor peacefully.

A BIRTHING MOMENT . . .

"One of the strongest memories from my birth was the calmness I felt as soon as Teresa arrived. And also that she always knew what I needed. I never had to ask. She even knew when I needed a fresh voice, and backed off while the midwife encouraged me to hold on without the epidural. I love her for that." —Patricia, Georgia

housework, cooking meals, running errands, and caring for older children. She may attend to a mother on bed-rest or help a mother with an uncomplicated pregnancy. Antepartum doulas also may provide lists of local resources, lend out books or informational videos, teach one-on-one childbirth education classes, practice relaxation techniques with the mother, or give the expectant mother a much-needed massage.

## LABOR DOULA

A labor doula helps a mother cope with labor pains and helps her have a pleasant birth experience, whether the mother wants to give birth normally, with medication, or is planning a c-section. She may meet with the mother before the birth to discuss the mother's expectations and her various options for labor. She helps the mother relax and feel confident, provides massage, and assists with laboring and pushing positions. The doula also helps the father participate in the birth to the extent that he feels comfortable. Some labor doulas take photographs, videotape the birth, or write a birth story.

## POSTPARTUM DOULA

A postpartum doula supports a new mother and family after the birth. She may help the new mother by doing light housework, cooking healthful meals for the family, entertaining the newborn's older siblings, or demonstrating newborn baby care, like bathing the baby or helping with breastfeeding. The doula may come every day for a few hours, a few times a week, or just provide support on the first day home. Some doulas will help care for the baby at night so the mother can rest in between late-night feedings.

> "[My doula] was able to anticipate my needs and questions and yet maintain a comfortable distance when I needed moments alone. She enabled me to manage my pain myself rather than relying on medication. When I did have to get an epidural for an unplanned c-section, she was wonderful at making me understand that I had not failed. She almost acted as an interpreter to my family when it came to what was going on in my mind." —Kathy, Texas

The majority of doulas have personal experience with pregnancy, birth, and motherhood, though a few are childless. There are several doula organizations that provide training, continuing education, referrals, and support for professionals. Doulas come in all shapes and sizes, from stay-at-home moms to retired business professionals, from women in their twenties to seasoned grandmothers. What they all have in common is a love for new motherhood and a desire to make pregnancy and childbirth the celebratory experience it is meant to be.

Nonmedical labor support is not a new idea. While professional doulas started to become popular in the United States in the 1990s, other cultures have always included nonmedical labor support. In a review of 128 developing countries, all but one provided women with the type of support a doula can offer. (Klaus M., Kennell J., Klaus P., 1993)

# Commonly Asked Questions

Q. What's the difference between a doula and a midwife?

A. A midwife is a trained medical professional. The midwife provides prenatal care and attends to the delivery. Midwives can assess fetal heart tones, check cervical dilation, watch for and treat complications of birth, and give medical advice. A doula does not perform any medical services and does not help with the actual birth. To put it bluntly, a doula works with the mother from the waist up, while the midwife primarily attends to the mother from the waist down.

Q. What kind of training do doulas receive?

A. Because there are no limits set on who can call themselves a doula and practice as one, training and experience varies. Most doulas, though, are either certified by a doula organization or have training that is similar to those that have completed the certification process. This usually includes reading several books on pregnancy and childbirth and, in some programs, completing book reports or exams. The doula may also attend a training session, usually a two- or three-day workshop. If she can't attend a workshop in person, some organizations provide videotaped training. She may be required to attend childbirth education, breastfeeding, or infant care

"For my third birth, I hired a homebirth midwife and planned to have all of my doula friends there to support me, and my kids to just be present. I really wanted to have an experience like the ones I had read about in tribal cultures. I wanted to be surrounded by women and encouraged by them. I wanted to be queen for a day and to only feel love when I looked around the room."
—Lucky, Wisconsin

"My mom was [at my baby's birth]. Believe me, I wanted my mommy there! But that was really her first/only birth that she witnessed. She was gassed and I was a forceps delivery—so she missed me coming out. When I was born, she was left alone in the maternity ward and no one, not even her mom or husband, was allowed to be with her. That was the era when you did not question the system. And she would not have the ability to challenge anything on my behalf."
—Lorraine, Michigan

classes as an observer. She must attend actual births as a doula, usually three to six, before she can be certified. Then, she may need to turn in evaluations from the parents, doctors, or nurses that were present at the births.

Q. I met a doula who called herself a *montrice*. What does that mean, exactly?

A. A montrice is a doula who also is trained to provide medical care, usually the kind of care a nurse provides. A nurse or midwife who is also trained as a doula may call herself a montrice when working in the role of a professional labor assistant.

## Why Doulas Are Needed in Our Modern Society

The need for doulas, both during labor and in the postpartum period, has never been greater. When childbirth moved from the home to the hospital in the early 1900s, women lost many of their freedoms and rights: The right to shout out during labor ("Please, not so loud, others will be bothered!"); the right to give birth in any position; the right to move around and walk during labor; the right to have one's family, friends, or husband in the room; and even the right to birth without the use of pain medications.

It wasn't until the 1960s and 1970s that the Lamaze movement began, and slowly, women started demanding their right to give birth normally. And they did have to fight. Doctors did not have any interest in dealing with someone who was "out of control." Birth was viewed as a medical event, not a celebration of life or a passage into motherhood, and the pressure of labor pains was viewed as a mistake of nature that needed to be fixed.

Since then, hospitals have started to provide women more rights and freedoms during labor. They are permitted by most hospitals to move around during labor, to have their partners and family with them, and to give birth with or without medication. Some hospitals allow laboring women to drink fluids in moderation. Unfortunately, with the exception of having the father or family in the room, hospitals rarely encourage women to exercise these rights.

Birth has become so "medicalized" that many view childbirth outside of the hospital environment as dangerous or risky. Those who choose to give birth at home or in a birthing center with a midwife need to defend their choices, usually being accused of "risking their life and their baby's life." A close look at statistics, though, shows that for healthy pregnant women, choosing to birth with a trained midwife outside of the hospital is just as safe, if not safer, than birthing in a hospital. (Springer and Weel, 1996)

"Twenty-six and 23 years ago, with the births of my first two sons, we were just happy to have Lamaze classes (that were taught in people's homes) and to find a doctor willing to go along with my Lamaze training. Doulas weren't the issue then. Husbands in the delivery room, birth without unnecessary medication, no strapping down on the delivery table, demand feeding—those were the big issues." —Barbara, Michigan

DID YOU KNOW?

In the 1950s, more than 40% of women gave birth outside of a hospital.

In 1999, less than 2% of women gave birth outside of a hospital.

Source: Statistics from the Center for Disease Control

Subconsciously, or consciously, the laboring mother may consider her labor contractions "dangerous" or feel that something is wrong. High anxiety may slow down labor, which may lead to medical interventions such as the use of oxytocin or other drugs, epidural block, or cesarean section. (L. Campero et al., 1998, 396)

"I actually did not want my mother at my birth, I just felt like she did not understand my desire for a natural birth and would be too negative and worried about every little thing to be a positive influence. My mother-in-law also doesn't understand the natural childbirth thing; she had planned cesareans for both of her children." —Lori, Florida

While childbirth is hard work, and the pressure and intensity does become great as labor progresses, fear and anxiety tend to magnify the pain. Magnified pain leads to more fear, into more pain, and the cycle continues, until the mother, hopefully, receives proper support or is given medication.

This is where the doula comes in. Doulas view pregnancy and childbirth as a natural process. They trust in the woman's body to birth her baby, and they respect a woman's individual way of laboring—whether she plans to use medication or not. At the same time, they are familiar with the medical procedures that are sometimes needed to help a mother and child give birth safely.

### 🐦 A BIRTHING MOMENT . . .

"After 38 hours of hard labor, including more than 10 hours of back labor, I was ready to give up. I was not progressing; my cervix was only 8 centimeters dilated. My doula told me that no matter what, I was going to be holding a beautiful baby in my arms in the next few hours. My doula turned up the lights and put some upbeat music on the radio. She told me it was time to have this baby and I could do it. We started to chant 'Rock the baby out! Rock the baby out!' as I rocked back and forth on the toilet. The change in the atmosphere and my husband's, my mother's, and my doula's encouragement made the difference. I became fully dilated and pushed the baby out in less than an hour." —Kari, California

Having someone present who trusts in the birth process, who wants nothing more than for the mother to have a positive birth experience and, at the same time, understands that there is a place and time for medical interventions, will radiate confidence onto the laboring woman. This will help stop the fear and anxiety cycle that so often spirals out of control. The doula can also help lessen the guilt that some mothers feel

"I would not have felt comfortable having a family member act as a doula because I felt like I would have to put on a show for them, 'be nice,' etc. With my doula, I did not worry if I got upset or vomited. She was paid to be there just like my doctor and the nurses." —Carrie, Florida

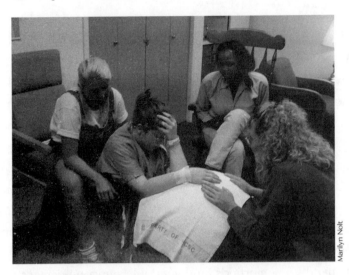

FIGURE 1.2.  Surrounded by her friends and doula,
a mother concentrates during a contraction.

when their birth plans do not go "perfectly," whether they wanted to give birth normally and needed an epidural, or when an emergency c-section is performed.

Some women want to use their mother, sister, or other female friend for support during labor. Most likely, their relative or friend does not possess the knowledge or skills to provide the best support. A doula has received training and has experience coaching women during labor. Plus, a mother or sister might find it difficult to remain objective and calm, and the laboring mother needs to be surrounded by confidence, not worry or pity.

For many families, having a mother or other female relative present for the birth is just not realistic. According to the United States Census Bureau, approximately 43 million Americans moved in the year 1999. Rarely do young families live in the same town they grew up in. This is also a reason that postpartum doulas are becoming more popular. The new mother may not have family or close friends that can help her.

When I became pregnant with my second child, a friend recommended that I have an experienced mother act as my birth coach. I hesitated for a variety of reasons. Would I feel intimidated by her or self-conscious around her? What would she think about my birth choices? And my biggest question was, would it really make a difference? Would it be worth the trouble and effort of finding a qualified doula? My birthing experience—and the research we'll discuss in the chapter 2— suggests that it is indeed worth the effort.

"I live 500 miles away from family and close friends, so I could not plan on my mother or one of my sisters or a close friend being in the labor and delivery room with me. . . . Although my husband would be there, I thought it would be invaluable to have someone in there who had been through a natural birth before."
—Michelle, North Carolina

PART TWO

# The Labor
# Doula

CHAPTER 2

# The Research
# on Labor Doulas

Don't skip this chapter! Perhaps you suffer from math pho-
bia or find research studies irrelevant to your situation. I've done my
best not to include unnecessary numbers or information and have
tried to present only the most interesting research studies. So please,
continue on. I suspect that you'll be pleasantly surprised.

## Studies and Testimonials

Information is power. Understanding how doulas improve the birth
experience can help you appreciate the need for labor support, boost
your confidence in your decision to have one, and enable you to encourage other women to use the services of a doula. Perhaps your
friend won't be impressed by your birth story or care to hear your
personal opinion on doulas. But she may be interested if you tell her
that doulas decrease the chance of interventions like episiotomies
and forceps deliveries.

From a professional standpoint, the research on doulas provides
guidance to hospitals and physicians. Several medical organizations
encourage the use of doulas, basing their decision on the research.

The American Academy of Family Physicians encourages the use of doulas because doulas decrease the need for pain medications, which in turn increases breastfeeding success rates. The American College of Obstetricians and Gynecologists encourages the use of doulas because their use lowers cesarean section rates in hospitals. Other organizations that encourage the use of doulas include the World Health Organization, the Medical Leadership Council of Washington, D.C., the nonprofit Institute for Healthcare Improvement in Boston, and the Society of Obstetricians and Gynecologists of Canada. (Jukelevics, 2002)

# Understanding the Research

When reviewing these studies, keep in mind that the women did not interview or choose who their labor support person would be. They also did not meet with the doula before or after the birth. If randomly assigned doulas improve the birth experience, imagine how much more improvement occurs when the mother can interview and choose a doula, speaking with her about the birth and her desires before labor begins. Though different people, in different hospitals, conducted the studies, they all followed these general guidelines:

**Healthy mothers.**  Only women who had normal, healthy pregnancies were eligible. High-risk patients were not included.

**Randomized trials.**  Whenever a healthy mother was admitted into the hospital where research was taking place, she was asked if she would like to participate in a study on the use of labor companions. She was told she might or might not receive labor support from another woman. If the mother agreed to participate, she was randomly assigned to either the doula or no doula group.

### 🐾 A BIRTHING MOMENT . . .

"I had been having contractions about 5 to 6 minutes apart for awhile, but I wasn't too concerned yet. I took a warm bath and was coping fairly well by breathing through each contraction, so I decided to try going to bed. As soon as I lied down, I had a very painful contraction—far worse than any previous one. I couldn't move or talk and felt like I couldn't even breathe. As soon as it stopped, I caught my breath and changed positions, thinking that might help. It didn't. The next one was just as bad with almost no break between them. I called for my husband and clung desperately to my birth ball. My husband timed the contractions—they were lasting 1½ to 2 minutes each with almost no break. "This is not how it's supposed to happen!" I thought. We called Terri immediately. We told her we thought it was time. She agreed to meet us and then asked how I was feeling. I said, "A little shaky, and a little scared." I started to cry. Thinking that I was only at the beginning, and it was already this bad, I was more terrified of labor than I had been during my entire pregnancy. If there was ever a time that I honestly didn't think I could do it, it was then. Terri just talked to me very calmly and reassured me that things would be all right. Hearing her calm, confident voice helped me regain my composure and got me through what was probably my most frightening moment." —Paula, Georgia

**Doula support.** The doulas were to provide emotional, physical, and informational support to the laboring woman from the time she was assigned up until the delivery. The doulas did not meet the women prior to admission, and they did not provide any postpartum support. In some studies, the doulas were lay midwives or nurses, and in other studies, the doulas were laywomen with no medical background.

# Positive Birth Experience

You will never forget the birth of your child. You will remember what you were doing that day and where you were when you first thought, "I think this is it." And you will remember how you felt during and after the birth. According to the latest research, your chance of having positive memories is higher if a doula supports you during labor and delivery.

A research team led, by Dr. Nancy P. Gordon of Kaiser Permanente's Division of Research discovered that women are more likely to rate their birth experience as "good" if a doula attends to them. The mothers who had the support of a doula were more likely to feel that they coped well with labor and to feel childbirth had a positive effect on their feelings as a woman and on their perception of physical strength and performance. See table 2.1 for the exact percentages. (Gordon et al., 1998)

"I was extremely proud of myself after I gave birth. I remember feeling relief and joy and a power I didn't know I possessed." —Erin, California

Another study concurs with Dr. Gordon's research. This unique study, led by Dr. Lourdes Campero, in Mexico, conducted in-depth interviews with the mothers. While it is impossible to measure the findings in an analytic way, the research gives us a good idea of how a doula improves the birthing experience.

In this study, women were asked to express in their own words how they felt the medical staff treated them; how they perceived medical information, routines, and interventions; how they experi-

| TABLE 2.1. | | |
| --- | --- | --- |

### How mothers rated their birth experience with or without a doula

| | Doula | No Doula |
| --- | --- | --- |
| Rated birth experience as good | 82.5% | 67.4% |
| Felt they coped well with labor | 46.8% | 28.3% |
| Felt labor had positive effect on them | | |
| as a woman | 58.0% | 43.7% |
| Perceived their bodies as strong | 58.0% | 41.0% |

Source: Gordon, Walton, McAdam, Derman, Gallitero, and Garrett,

California, 1998. *Obstetrics & Gynecology 93, no. 3* (1999): 422–26.

enced labor and their self-perceptions during the process; and how they felt about having a labor companion. It's important to note that those who did not have a doula present were alone, without husband or family members.

The women who did not have a doula were less likely to express themselves freely when asked how they felt the medical staff treated them. While most of them said they had little or no communication with the staff, and a few said the staff was rough with them during examinations, they all said they were "grateful" for the care they received. However, the women who received support from a doula were forthright about the way they were treated, whether they felt anger or gratitude. "Such extremes," Dr. Campero writes, "indicate how being taken into account made it easier for them to express themselves, and gave them the feeling of having some rights."

The women who were supported by a doula found it easier to ask questions of the medical staff, even when the hospital was busy.

The doulas encouraged the women to ask questions, and when the mothers did not ask the medical staff, they talked to their doulas about options and fears. The group that did not receive support from a doula asked very few questions, and when they did ask questions, they were often given pat answers like, "There is nothing to worry about."

During labor, the group without a doula lost track of time and did not know if they were getting closer to the birth or what they should expect next. The moms that did have a doula were more aware of the various stages of labor and knew that as time progressed, they were getting closer to the birth.

Most important, those birthing with the help of a doula had a more positive attitude toward themselves and felt that their hard work is what brought the new baby into this world. They felt more in control and had higher self-esteem. Conversely, the women who were not supported by a doula felt like passive participants in the birth. They viewed the last moments of labor as a series of medical interventions that finally led to the birth of the baby, and the women gave the doctors all the credit. (Campero et al., 1998)

In both Dr. Campero's study and Dr. Gordon's study, the women who were supported by a doula said they would like a doula to accompany them the next time they give birth. In addition, those who

> "[The doula] primarily reminded my husband and me of things we would have otherwise forgotten. For instance, what questions to ask to be fully informed, which was especially helpful after I was diagnosed with preeclampsia. I really knew nothing about it, its treatment options, the risks of going untreated, etc. Our doula acted as a silent advocate; she talked to us and then let my husband and/or I talk to the nurses and doctors."
> —Michelle, North Carolina

A BIRTHING MOMENT . . .

"Just as I was entering active labor, we had just come in from a walk, and she suggested we put on some music. I had made a special CD of happy music for early labor. It was very upbeat, and as we listened, I danced with my husband, leaning on him with my arms around his neck, and my doula stood behind me, dancing too, and rubbing my back. We were all singing, and it felt so joyous to me! It was like I had all the strength in the world to birth my baby!"
—Melanie, Washington

did not have a support person expressed the desire to have a doula if they have any more children.

# Reduced Need for Pain Medication

Women spend nine months of pregnancy doing whatever they can to avoid unnecessary drugs or toxins. They avoid cold and pain medicines and try to use safer alternatives. Some buy organic fruits and vegetables or avoid chemically-treated tap water. However, when labor begins, many women throw their concerns out the window and use drugs, without even trying for a normal birth. Who can blame them? Childbirth, like parenting, is hard work. Without proper support and a great deal of preparation, giving birth without drugs is difficult, to say the least!

Drugs used during childbirth affect the unborn child and carry risks to the mother. Narcotics can produce several negative side effects in the mother, including nausea, dizziness, blurred memory, depression, drowsiness, vomiting, and low blood pressure. Narcotics

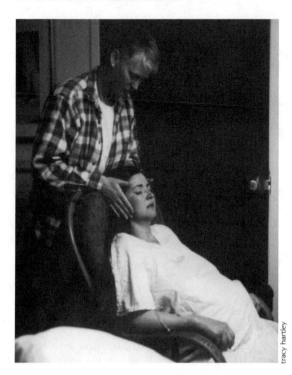

FIGURE 2.1. Doula tracy hartley of BestDoulas.com helps a mother maintain a state of deep relaxation, eliminating the need for pain medications.

are usually limited to early labor to avoid a groggy baby. In the new-born, narcotics can lead to fetal heart decelerations, inability to suck just after birth, or labored breathing. Sometimes, additional drugs are administered to the baby after birth to counteract side effects. (Eisenberg et al., 1996)

Epidurals are considered "safe," but, like any drug, they can negatively affect the mother and unborn child. Risks to the mother include spinal headaches, persistent back pain, incontinence, and a rare but real chance of irreversible nerve damage and paralysis. Studies on epidural use have shown an increased c-section rate, longer pushing stage, increased need for forceps or vacuum extraction, increased rate of episiotomies, and a higher risk of maternal fever. (England, P., Horowitz, R., 1998)

Contrary to popular belief, the drugs that are used in an epidural do pass through the placenta to the baby. One study showed that epidural use might interfere with the infant's instinctual breastfeeding behaviors and increase the baby's temperature. Newborns whose mothers used an epidural also cried more.

One research paper states, "The reason why the infants exposed to analgesia cried more is not known. Studies have shown that infant crying behavior contains different messages, such as hunger, pain, and distress. . . . A possible explanation is that infant crying can be a sign of frustration at not being able to suck the breast, when the instinct to reach out to the breasts is there. However, other effects cannot be ruled out." (Ransjö-Arvidson et al., 2001)

Of course, there is a time and place for medicated pain relief. Pain medication plays an important role in a birth that is unusually long, is augmented with induction medications, or is in any other way abnormal or unusually stressful for the mother. But in a normal birth, drugs should be avoided, or at the very least, delayed and used with caution.

"After 13 hours of labor, I chose to get an epidural. After about 6 hours, it stopped working on my lower abdomen, right where all the contractions were. The anesthesiologist tried to correct the problem, but to do that, he pumped me full of drugs—vial after vial after vial. Finally, after about 2 hours, it got back on track, but it really freaked me out that I had so many drugs in my system and my baby's system." —Jennifer, Wisconsin

Several research projects concluded that doulas help women avoid drugs during a normal birth. The most impressive study on doulas and the use of pain medication took place in a Houston hospital in 1991. This study had three groups. One group received support from a doula, another group received no doula support, and a third group had a woman sit silently in the room behind a curtain.

In the doula supported group, only 7.8 percent of the mothers requested an epidural. In the group that had a woman silently sit in the room, 22.6 percent of the women requested an epidural. Compare these two percentages with the group that had no support and no silent observer: 55.3 percent of the unsupported moms asked for an epidural. (Kennell et al., 1991) See table 2.2 for results from other studies.

> "I was induced, and by the time I hit 3 centimeters, I was in horrible pain. They gave me either Stadol or Demerol and Phenergan, and I feel that they gave me too much. I was drugged beyond belief and don't remember much of my labor or what happened afterwards. It was a horrible feeling." —Ashley, Alabama

Even if you think you'll need medication to cope with labor, a doula can help you avoid medication until you really need it. Research confirms that delaying an epidural can decrease the risk of a cesarean section. (England, P., Horowitz, R., 1998) A separate study showed that newborns had less trouble breastfeeding if the medication exposure was less than one hour, as opposed to several hours. (Crowell M., P. Hill, & S. Humenick, 1994)

# Breastfeeding and Bonding

To breastfeed a child is to give her a gift that is irreplaceable. Besides the nutritional superiority of breast milk, research has shown that breastfeeding raises IQ scores. (Mortensen, 2002) The release of the hormone prolactin during breastfeeding helps the mother feel calm and helps the baby sleep. This hormone also creates a unique bond be-

| TABLE 2.2. | | |
| --- | --- | --- |
| **Percentage of women who used an epidural or other pain medication during labor** | | |
| | Doula | No Doula |
| Kennell et al. | 7.8% | 55.3% |
| Hodnett et al. | 61.0% | 82.0% |
| Gordon et al. | 54.3% | 66.1% |

tween the mother and her baby. The American Academy of Pediatricians suggests that mothers breastfeed their babies for at least one year and yet, according to the World Health Organization, barely one in three infants are exclusively breastfed for the first four months of their life.

According to Dr. G. Hofmeyr of Johannesburg, South Africa, doula-supported mothers have a better chance of breastfeeding their children successfully. In his study, mothers who received doula support were more likely to be breastfeeding exclusively at six weeks postpartum and twice as likely to be feeding their infants on a flexible schedule. Mothers who were not supported were four times more likely to report problems with breastfeeding and three times as likely to be feeding their infants food other than breast

> "My husband and I took 20 hours of Bradley childbirth, were well prepared for what to expect, chose a good provider, and gave long and careful thought to our birth plan. But labor is work, painful, at times almost exhausting. Having constant, expert physical and emotional support through this process was irreplaceable!"
> —Stephanie, New Jersey

# Why I Chose Natural Childbirth

Six mothers share their reasons for choosing to birth without medication.

*Ruth:* "I wanted a natural childbirth because I felt it was the safest option for my child and me. After losing two babies to miscarriage, safety was my number one concern. However, I did try to have an open mind about the possibility of using pain relief if my birth experience did not go according to plan. Amazingly, we followed every step of our birth plan and I was able to have a water birth and a completely natural childbirth."

*Michelle:* "I wanted to give my baby the very best start in life. I took good care of myself during my pregnancy, so it followed for me that natural childbirth was the way to go. Why would I want to introduce something toxic (pain-relieving drugs) into my system after I had spent months and months avoiding anything that could potentially be harmful to the precious life growing inside of me? I wouldn't!"

*Trish:* "I chose natural childbirth because the process of birth is so unique. Delivering a new person into the world requires enormous strength, and I embraced the way my body knew just what to do. Although painful, I enjoyed being free of drugs and able to understand exactly what was happening at each stage. I wanted to experience it in its totality, to feel my body's power and to truly be one with nature in this experience."

*Dina:* "I had Pitocin with my first childbirth and the contractions were so hard and so close together that I couldn't use any breathing techniques to help control the pain. I felt completely out of control. I was determined to have a better experience with my second childbirth, so I hired a doula to help me with a natural birth."

## Why I Chose Natural Childbirth (*continued*)

*Karen:* "I did not want anyone putting a needle in my spine if it was not necessary.... I was able to stay home until I was 7 centimeters with my first and 8 centimeters with my second. I was very happy with my labor and delivery. I felt I was in control, and both of my girls arrived happy, healthy, and very alert."

*Monica:* "This is a strong statement but I am convinced that the epidural I got during labor caused me to need the c-section I had with my first baby. Basically, my baby got stuck and could not descend. I have not and will not *ever* get another epidural for labor. I have since had two great natural [vaginal] births!"

milk at six weeks of age. (Hofmeyr et al., 1991) For more details, see table 2.3.

It's important to mention that the doulas in this study did not provide any postpartum support. When asked by the researchers if they helped the mothers with breastfeeding, the doulas said they did not provide any specific information on breastfeeding or help with the infant's first meal. Pure emotional support during labor is what increased breastfeeding success.

The questionnaire asked the mothers who stopped breastfeeding why they choose to bottlefeed. Interestingly, 32 percent of the mothers who were not supported by a doula blamed lack of milk supply, compared to 13 percent of the doula-supported mothers. Is it possible that the mothers who were supported by a doula viewed their bodies as strong and capable, while the mothers who were not supported considered their bodies as deficient?

TABLE 2.3.

## Results of questionnaire at 6 weeks postpartum

|  | Doula | No Doula |
|---|---|---|
| Exclusively breastfeeding | 51.4% | 29.3% |
| On food other than milk | 17.6% | 53.3% |
| Has had feeding problems | 16.2% | 62.7% |
| Feeding on a flexible schedule | 81.1% | 46.7% |

Source: Hofmeyr, Nikodem, Wolman, Chalmers, and Kramer; 1991, South Africa.
*British Journal of Obstetrics and Gynaecology 98* (1991): 756–764.

"After the mess of all the drugs and interventions, [the doula and I] chatted about how the first breastfeeding attempt might not go so well but that my baby girl and I should at least get familiar with each other. She cleared the room, got both of us calm and situated, and my little champ and I had no problems breastfeeding."
—Anne, Texas

The women were also asked how they felt about motherhood. Of the doula-supported mothers, 44.6 percent said they found becoming a mother easy, as opposed to only 10.7 percent of the non-supported mothers. When asked if they were "managing the baby well," 90.5 percent of the doula-supported mothers said they were, compared to 65.3 percent of the nonsupported mothers.

Who's to say how an unsupported birth experience will affect a mother's view of herself and how much that will affect her ability to parent her newborn, or how it will affect her willingness to breastfeed her child?

# Top 10 Reasons to Hire a Labor Doula

1. You want to give birth normally, without the use of medication or unnecessary interventions.
2. You want someone who is experienced and trained to help manage your labor pain. (Epidurals are not administered immediately and sometimes do not work properly.)
3. You've heard about the research on doulas and want the benefit of having one present.
4. You want someone knowledgeable present at all times to ask questions and explain your options. (The nurses and doctors will be in and out of the room.)
5. You want someone to act as an advocate for your and your partner's wishes.
6. You've experienced a traumatic or negative birth with prior children.
7. You're a single mother or your partner is out of town (for example in the military service).
8. You're trying for a VBAC (vaginal birth after cesarean).
9. You want someone present who can provide physical or emotional support, if the father cannot be present or participate for religious reasons.
10. You want someone to help the father participate more fully in the birth, to take pictures or video, and to deal with family and friends.

Dr. Hofmeyr's research team wrote, "[W]e need to accept the premise that labor is a time of unique sensitivity to environmental factors, and that events and interactions during labor may have far-reaching psychological consequences. Given the fact that very few human experiences approach in intensity the levels of stress, anxiety, pain, exertion, and emotional tumult which occur during labor, this is not surprising." (Hofmeyr et al., 1991)

# Medical Interventions

A meta-analysis is a mathematical research method that allows integration of several statistical studies into one. A research team, led by Dr. Kathryn D. Scott, Dr. Gale Berkowitz, and Dr. Marshall Klaus, used meta-analysis to combine the findings of five different studies on doulas. What they concluded is just amazing.

> "[My doula] definitely helped me avoid a c-section. I labored on Pitocin for 36 hours. I was exhausted. If Tracy hadn't gotten in my face and told me to push like she did, I would have gone through all that labor for nothing and had a c-section. No one else in the room cared that much about seeing me avoid a c-section." —Erin, California

They found that continuous support from a doula reduces the requests for pain medication by 36 percent and reduces the need for oxytocin, a drug that speeds up labor, by 71 percent. They also found that labor is shortened an average of an hour and a half for doula-supported moms. In addition, they concluded that a mother who does not use a doula is twice as likely to have a cesarean section or forceps delivery. (Scott, Berkowitz, & Klaus; 1999) See table 2.4.

Take note that these studies took place in hospitals where intervention rates were generally high. Most were not allowed any companions in the labor room except the doula, and many women came from low-income backgrounds (hence, little or no childbirth education). Logically, a hospital or birth center that already has a low c-section rate will not see dramatic improvement when doulas are

TABLE 2.4.

# Meta-analysis of several doula studies

36% reduction in use of pain medications

51% reduction in c-sections

71% reduction in use of oxytocin

57% reduction in forceps deliveries

An average of 1 hour and 38 minutes shorter labor

Source: Scott, Berkowitz, & Klaus; 1999, California.
*American Journal of Obstetrics and Gynecology 180, No. 5* (1999): 1054–1059.

included on the birth team. And of course, some c-sections are necessary for a healthy mother and baby.

These findings are significant and are especially important for hospitals with high intervention rates. The Centers for Disease Control (CDC) published a report stating that birth by cesarean section has increased, and not decreased, despite a national effort to lower the percentages. According to the report, delivery by cesarean section dropped by 8 percent between 1991 and 1996, but then began to rise over the next three years. In 2000, 23 percent of births in the United States were cesarean sections—the highest rate since 1990. See table 2.5.

Dr. Fay Menacker and Sally C. Curtin write in the *National Vital Statistics Reports: Trends in Cesarean Birth and Vaginal Birth after Previous Cesarean:*

The fact that the rise has been widespread for women of all ages and races and for nearly all states supports the idea that there has been

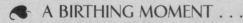

## A BIRTHING MOMENT . . .

"Her words really helped. It hurt a lot more than I expected. I thought there would be a lot more downtime for some reason. Like a cop hanging out at the donut shop waiting for crime to occur, I thought I'd be waiting for the baby to appear or at least waiting for when I have to start pushing! Silly, I know! So I was pretty over-whelmed with the pain at times. She told me lots of soothing things but also things like, this is our lot in life and it does hurt and most every woman gets through it, it'll be okay! Also when I considered an epidural, I said, "Georg'ann, tell me again why I don't want an epidural!" She had the know-how to run down the pros and cons for me during labor. My friends certainly could not have done that and I can't imagine an OB nurse having the time or patience to do it. I'm an academic; I needed to review the info again and again. The birth was medication-free, definitely due to Georg'ann's presence. I was very close to asking for pain meds and she, knowing my prefer-ence for natural birth, got me to hang in there." —Mary, California

a general change in the approach to childbirth in the United States. There continues to be considerable variation in cesarean and VBAC rates by state. In fact, one state achieved and a few states closely ap-proached the year 2000 objective of 15 per 100 births, while many states had rates that were at least 50 percent higher than the objec-tive. The pronounced disparities in state-specific cesarean rates per-sist even after differences in maternal age and birth order are considered. It is probable that these marked variations are related to local practice patterns. Research on strategies used by states that safely maintain a lower rate of cesarean births might assist those working toward a decreased rate. (Menacker and Curtin, 2001)

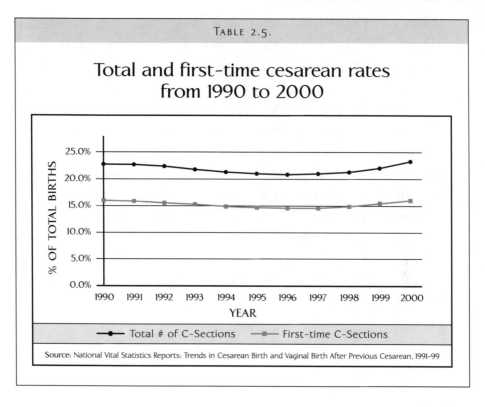

TABLE 2.5.

## Total and first-time cesarean rates from 1990 to 2000

Total # of C-Sections — First-time C-Sections

Source: National Vital Statistics Reports: Trends in Cesarean Birth and Vaginal Birth After Previous Cesarean, 1991–99

What is frightening about this statement is, it implies the high cesarean rates are not based on more high-risk pregnancies and births, but are the result of doctors' philosophies and hospital practices. (My personal advice: Find out what the c-section rate is at the hospital where you plan to give birth.)

As a response to the CDC's report, the American College of Obstetricians and Gynecologists

"My doula was there with me in the hospital from the beginning of the induction to see that I was informed about the risks and benefits of any procedures and most important, just to be there by my side. Her presence kept us calm and better able to work with the labor instead of against it." —Alissa, Illinois

published a paper with suggestions to help reduce the c-section rate. One of their suggestions was, "The continuous presence of nurses or other trained individuals who provide comfort and support to women in labor may lead to lower rates." Essentially, they suggest using a doula, and many hospitals throughout the nation are starting doula programs and encouraging their use.

A downfall of some hospital doula programs is they fail to provide "continuous" support to the laboring mother, usually because of shift changes. The research we examined by Dr. Scott, Dr. Berkowitz, and Dr. Klaus showed that continuous support from a doula has a stronger effect than intermittent support. If you plan to use a doula from a hospital program, you may want to ask if the same doula will be able to stay with until you give birth. If not, seriously consider hiring a private doula.

## CHAPTER 3

# Comfort and Services

Now you're familiar with the research, and you have a general idea of what doulas do. Let's focus on how a doula—by providing informational, emotional, and physical support—can help you achieve the amazing outcomes we've discussed.

Every doula is different, as is every mother. What helps one mom relax may make another mother tense. When you meet with your doula, tell her what you think you'll like, and she'll help you understand your options. When reading this chapter you may want to jot down the ideas you'd like to discuss with your doula.

## Informational Support

One important aspect of your doula's job is to provide you with information, before, during, and after childbirth. After your initial interview with the doula, you may meet with her two or three more times before the birth. During these prenatal meetings, your doula will listen to your thoughts and fears, help you find information on questions you have, and discuss your desires and options for childbirth.

🐦 A BIRTHING MOMENT . . .

"My epidural had completely worn off and I started crying and feeling totally out of control. The nurse came in and checked me and the baby's head was right there ready to come on out. I remember my doula grabbing my face as I was really starting to lose it and saying, 'Come on, keep it together, don't lose it, look at me! Deep low moans, Jessica.' My baby only took about six minutes to come out and while I was keeping my eyes shut and pushing, my doula said, 'Open your eyes and look at your baby boy!' I finally opened my eyes and for the first time watched my baby come out. It was absolutely amazing watching my baby slide out of me. I never would have looked had she not reminded me to do so." —Jessica, Georgia

ATTITUDES

Usually, the first meeting with your doula will be spent talking about your thoughts on birthing.

"I try to demystify labor," says Cyndi Whitwell of California, a doula who has attended over two hundred births. "If it is a first-time mom, I explain labor as a journey, a process that starts at point A and ends up at point B. There are highs and lows to it, but it is a do-able process. It is not some big monster you have to tackle."

Your doula may offer books, videos, or pamphlets on pregnancy, childbirth, and postpartum topics. "I started giving away birth balls to every client about two years ago," says Whitwell. A birth ball is a physical therapy ball, usually 26 inches in diameter (see figure 3.1). "I show them eight positions to use it with, but I especially empha-size the hands-and-knees position over the ball and ask them to as-

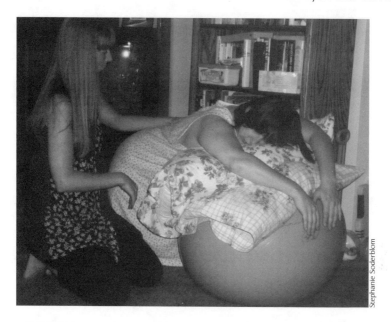

FIGURE 3.1. A mother uses a birth ball with pillows to support herself.

sume this position every day for about ten to fifteen minutes. Since doing this, I have really seen a huge decrease in back labor."

### BIRTH PLANS/WISH LISTS

Your doula will also help you develop a birth plan, if you want one, and discuss your various options for labor.

"For those who have not made any decisions yet," explains Uta from South Carolina, a doula since 1995, "I will offer them scenarios and possibilities, choices they may have, along with the pros and cons of each, so that they can see what they might be comfortable with, what they might find appealing."

Doulas also provide support via telephone or e-mail, starting when you sign the contract up until a few weeks postpartum. To get the most out of your doula, ask questions. Don't be afraid to call to

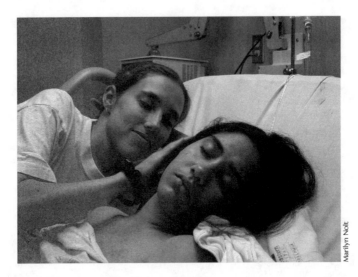

FIGURE 3.2: With a doula at her side,
this mom prepares to birth her baby.

discuss your thoughts or concerns. Most doulas are on-call 24-hours a day for two weeks before and after your due date.

Be aware that there is quite a bit of controversy surrounding birth plans. Some feel that birth plans are an important part of getting the birth experience a mother wants. Others feel that birth plans set a couple up for failure. Since labor is unpredictable, and a birth plan cannot account for every possible scenario, the mother and father may feel that they failed if the birth does not go according to the "plan."

"I suggest that they not use the phrase 'birth plan' but instead make a 'wish list'," says Uta, "or a description of what her/their 'ideal birth' would be like. I think such a list is an essential tool for communication for the woman with her partner, for the woman with her caregivers, and for the woman/couple with her doula."

Here are some tips on writing your wish list:

- *Talk about your options and thoughts with your partner and doula first.* If you don't know what to expect or are not aware of the many options, then writing a wish list will not be productive. Uta suggests "sitting down and thinking about the various possibilities and wishes, discussing and explaining and exploring them with the members of [your] birth team." Candid discussion will help you figure your plans out better and help your support team understand better what you want.

- *Keep your wish list short, no more than one page.* Nurses and doctors are very busy, and anything longer than one page probably will not be read. Your doula can help you focus on the most important aspects of your birth desires and help you write a plan that is concise and to the point.

- *Avoid negative language.* Try to use positive statements. For example, instead of "I do not want medication; please do not offer me drugs," you can write, "I want to give birth normally without medication. I will ask for medication if I need it."

> "I met with my doula a few times before birth, but we spoke on the phone frequently because I had a lot of false labor. When it was discovered my child was engaging posterior, she sent us information on how to get him to turn into an anterior position, and it worked."
> —Peri, Florida

- *Add a personal touch to your birth wish list.* You're one of several patients, and a unique-looking birth wish list will help the nurses and doctors distinguish yours from others. Use colored paper and readable fonts. Add a picture of yourself (or you and your partner), or a clip-art photo.

- *Review your birth wishes with your doctor or midwife.* "I tell them to just ask if there is anything on it that won't happen at this particular facility," says Whitwell. "If the doctor says,

'Sounds reasonable' or 'This is standard, there's no problem with your desires,' then we all feel comfortable that this doctor or hospital will be working with us to provide the birth the couple desires."

- *Make sure your doula has a copy of the birth wish list.* "A written birth preference list also helps me advocate better," explains Uta. "It clearly shows the mother's preferences and that I am not following some kind of personal agenda when reminding staff of her wishes."

- Bring *multiple copies of the wish list to the hospital or birth center.* This is especially important if your doctors or midwives practice in a group setting. The doctor who admits you to the hospital may not be the one that helps with the delivery, and the nurses will most likely change shifts while you are there. If the mother brings a written copy of her birth wish list with her, "she will not need to verbally inform every new nurse caring for her, but instead she or her partner can just pull out another copy of her list and hand it over," says Uta.

- *Use the Internet to help you write your wish list.* A good website to try is http://epregnancy.com/tools/birthplan.htm.

## PAIN MANAGEMENT

During labor, doulas provide information on pain management techniques, risks and benefits to certain procedures, and options that the couple may not have considered. "There are many tools one can use in labor—medication is only one of them," explains Whitwell. "There are position changes, hydration, change of lighting in the room, change of smells such as with massage oils, massage, water whether in a tub or shower, heat or cold, movement, etc."

Often the nurses or doctors may recommend a certain procedure they'd like to try, like rupturing the bag of waters, or they may want to start using labor augmentation medications, like Pitocin. Your doula can help you understand what your options are and explain the risks or benefits.

"When [the couple is] in the heat of labor and a decision has to be made, I try to give them many options," says Whitwell. "If you do this, this might happen. If you do this, this might happen. Then when they make a decision, I verbally support it if the mom feels confident in her decision. If she felt informed and it is informed consent, then that is the whole purpose behind 'empowering' a woman to take charge of her own birth. That is my job, to empower her to believe in her decisions."

A doula does not, however, give medical advice. "If they are asking me a question that needs to be answered by a doctor, I always encourage them to call their medical provider," assures Whitwell. "I tell them there are no 'stupid' questions if it is a concern to them."

> "I lost count of how many times my doula and I spoke on the phone; some conversations lasted over an hour. She supported me before labor by helping me sort through my feelings from my previous birth, briefed me on what to expect from my attempt at a VBAC and the things we could expect at the hospital due to my previous c-section." —Lori, Nebraska

## ADVOCACY

Advocacy is part of informational support. "I think that the best way to advocate is to inform," says DeeDee Farris-Folkerts of Missouri, who has been a doula for over seven years. "So many people believe that it is all out of their hands, that what the doctor or midwife says, goes. Not so! Question everything."

Farris-Folkerts recommends her clients ask the BRAND questions whenever an intervention or action is being suggested. What are the Benefits of this particular procedure? What are the Risks? What are our Alternatives? What happens if we do Nothing? And

"There were a few times when I was just too tired to think to ask questions and the doula helped remind me. For example, when the nurse put in an internal monitor to monitor the contractions, she wanted to put in a fetal scalp monitor. The doula reminded me to ask why she wanted to put in the fetal scalp monitor. The nurse said it was not because of the baby's heartbeat, which was fine, but because if she put in the fetal scalp monitor she would not have to keep adjusting the belt on my stomach. I was then able to make an informed decision and refuse the fetal scalp monitor because it was not needed. The nurse just wanted to use it for her convenience." —Carrie, Florida

please give us time alone to think about our options and make a Decision.

"I remind parents that it is their responsibility to speak up for themselves," explains Farris-Folkerts. "I am not there to speak for them, only to inform them, let them know their options, and to support them in their decisions. Every once in a while, when a doctor or nurse is stating something that they intend to do, and the parents seem a bit lost, I will cue them by saying, 'Do you have any questions about this?' This reminds them to use BRAND."

# Emotional Support

You will experience a wide range of emotions during this special time. Your feelings may fluctuate between fear and tranquility, extreme pain and then calming ecstasy, or tears and hopelessness, followed by joy and awe. A doula can help you experience those

**A BIRTHING MOMENT . . .**

"I was standing over the bathroom sink, having vomited and then brushed my teeth, and I looked up into the mirror. There was a woman looking out at me I had never seen before. A primal, strong, intense mother. DeeDee, who was standing behind me rubbing my back, said 'Look at you. Look how strong and beautiful you are. You can do this. You are doing this.' It was a moment." —Koren, Missouri

feelings within a safe context. She can help you remain calm, or conversely, provide the security you need to let yourself "lose control."

> "She was so confident and knowledgeable, and that alone helped me to relax."
> —Jennifer, Florida

### RELAXATION

One part of emotional support is helping you relax. When you relax, you work with your body, not against it. This lessens painful sensations and encourages labor along.

"The only breathing I recommend to a laboring woman is normal breathing patterns: nice, slow, abdominal breathing," says Jane Cruice of Pennsylvania, a doula who has attended women in birth centers, hospitals, and at home. "I believe that any patterned breathing is more likely to hyperventilate the mother, and sometimes make her more stressed out. It's difficult to be stressed out when you are focusing on nice abdominal breaths going in and out."

Visualizations may help you remain calm during childbirth. Some women imagine a rose that is blossoming, or they picture their cervix opening, while their baby moves further down the birth canal.

Others prefer to turn their focus away from what's happening at the birth, remembering a peaceful moment from their lives. Your doula can help by speaking to you in a low, soft voice or, for example, she may remind you to "picture the rose blossoming."

"When she is dealing inside with frustration and it shows by the head starting to shake in a 'no' direction, I start giving her reassurance that all is well," explains doula Cyndi Whitwell, "All she has to deal with is the moment—what does she need to do in this moment? Does she need to change positions, relax a certain muscle, slow her breathing, take a drink of something? This all plays into her emotional level at the time . . . giving her ideas that makes her feel she is still in control of herself."

"Teresa had a mock labor class for all of her clients, which helped me face my fears about birth. Up to this point I had let my fears sort of simmer below the level of my awareness, and I just felt apprehension. After that class, I e-mailed Teresa with my list of top 10 fears about birth and we discussed them."
—Patricia, Georgia

A doula can also help you work through the feelings from previous births. "Before the labor I emphasize that this will not be the same birth," says Whitwell. "I say, 'You are not in the same place in your life, this is not the same baby, your body is not the same.' And [during labor,] I try to point out the positive parts about this experience—it's going more quickly, you are so relaxed, baby is looking great, here's a position you may not have tried before, etc."

SPIRITUALITY

Spirituality is another important part of emotional support. "I believe every birth is a spiritual birth," says Cruice. "I had a Muslim woman client laboring in a hospital and in order to help her have time to pray I would 'guard' the door so that she wouldn't have any intrusions during her prayers, which she ended up needing to do three times during her labor.

"Also, at the actual moment of birth she requested silence in the room—and got it!" explains Cruice. "What I found most interesting about this situation was how much more cooperation we received when it was for 'religious' reasons than when I have been with clients who just wished to be left alone to labor quietly in their room because it would help them labor more effectively. Those clients' wishes are often not taken as seriously."

> "Both my second and third labors and births were short (from one to three hours), and even so, I could not have done it without Heather. I'm a religious person, and although I know that G-d is with me every time I birth, I feel an extra blessing when He allows me to have Heather there too."—Sara, Massachusetts

### THE ENVIRONMENT

Maintaining the birthing environment is another way doulas help moms cope. The doula may dim the lights, play soft music, or keep family members occupied. She may help straighten up the room, make sure you have enough pillows, fetch ice chips or pat a cool wash cloth on your face. She'll be there if your partner needs to leave the room, making sure you are never left alone—unless that is what you want.

# Physical Support

While I personally do not like people touching me during labor, I felt relieved when my doula dabbed a cool washcloth on my face during transition. My doula helped support me in my pushing position, so I could focus my energy on birthing my baby. Doulas provide physical support and pain management techniques through a variety of

"She brought water or juice for me as needed, made sure I had extra pillows, etc. She brought a hot pack filled with rice and went to the nurse's microwave to heat it for me. I had selected some aromatherapy scents that she brought to me upon request. I wanted to hold a particular object I'd brought while contracting in the labor pool and she put it in my hand. In addition, when the birth was over and we were transitioning into the mother/baby ward, my doula cleaned up all of our personal items and repacked them in our bag for us, which was a great relief." —Lynn, North Carolina

actions: massage, acupressure, providing counterpressure, supporting the mother in different positions.

"I recently attended a client whose epidural was, for a while, so concentrated on one side that her leg kept sliding off the bed, and it made it impossible for her to sleep," explains Elizabeth Lott, a doula in Massachusetts. "I sat in a rocker next to the bed and arranged myself so that the sole of my foot rested against the sole of hers, and stayed that way for a couple hours so she could get some sleep. Who says you don't need a doula if you have an epidural?!"

POSITIONS

Your doula may suggest different movements or positions, and then help support you, especially during contractions. Some women labor while sitting on the toilet and others enjoy standing in a shower. Walking lessens the pain for some women and may speed up labor.

"I strongly believe in the gate pain control theory, which basically says that the more stimuli you can introduce to the brain at once, the better the pain signal to the brain is broken up," explains Heather Kleber, a doula and certified childbirth educator from Colorado. "In practical terms, this means that I'll have my clients doing several things at once—perhaps moaning through contractions while rocking on the birth ball, with music on and essential oils burning, or squatting during a contraction while I do a double-hip squeeze on mom, and dad is using paced breathing with mom during her contraction."

## ACUPRESSURE

Some doulas are knowledgeable in the science of acupressure. "Spleen 6, a point on the inside of the lower leg about four finger widths (the mom's fingers, not mine) above the ankle, and just behind the tibia, is often effective in establishing a good pattern of contractions when mom is having contractions that are disorganized and ineffective," explains doula Elizabeth Lott.

Other pressure points in the body are said to release endorphins when stimulated. Endorphins are the body's natural pain killers.

"I have mom hold a small comb in each hand, and with contractions she squeezes the combs, pressing the teeth into these creases," says Lott. "A few moms have found this very helpful . . . Other moms to whom I have suggested this founded it distracting in a negative way. As with any labor support technique, it works for some, and not for others."

> "During the pushing phase I remember her being on one side of me and my husband on the other side supporting my arms and sides. I was sitting on a birthing stool and she was right there cheering me on." —Kim, Mexico

## MASSAGE

Massage is another tool doulas use to help support their clients. The doula may massage her client's feet, arms, or back. She may rub her

"[My doula] gave me a massage on my lower back and my hands. This helped me focus on something other than the pain. Once the Pitocin was started, I began to really work through my contractions. I was moving constantly trying to get away from the pain. Teresa seemed to know what I needed before I had to ask. So until about noon, I went from my birth ball, to dancing with my husband, to leaning on the bed. At this point, I wasn't able to handle my contractions very well. I just couldn't get away from my back pain. The nurse checked me and told us that I was still dilated about the same as I had been when my midwife checked me that morning. That was my lowest point. I began sobbing. Teresa and Erik worked so hard for me during this time. Teresa sat back to back with me on the bed and would push into my back with hers during contractions; in between I would doze. I was so thankful for the rest in between."
—Patricia, Georgia

temples or brush her hair. *Effleurage,* or gliding the hands gently over the skin, can help.

"Intention is an important aspect of effective touch," says Lott. "When I touch or massage a laboring mom, I'm doing more than laying my hands on her, or soothing her muscles. My intention is totally focused on her, my mind's eye visualizes her path, and my energy flows to her through my hands."

When a mother is experiencing back labor, a doula can provide counterpressure, or use her body or hands to push against the mother's back, helping to relieve the pain.

"I attended one labor where the mom had nasty back labor, and nothing we did helped except really strong counterpressure to her low back," explains Lott. "Her husband, the midwife, and I all switched off providing the pressure, with mom in a variety of positions, until our arms were exhausted, and even at maximum force she still said it was not enough pressure. Finally, with mom side-lying on the bed, her husband knelt on the floor, leaned in, and did the counterpressure with the top of his head! Mom said, 'That's it! Don't stop that!' Dad was able to hold the position, and did so until mom was ready to push."

## AFTER THE BIRTH

Usually, your doula will leave within an hour or so of the birth. She may then visit you in the hospital or call to ask how you're doing and if you have any questions. Most doulas will meet with you a few weeks after the birth to talk.

"I love to hear what they have to say about their birth experience," says Kim Govekar, a doula in Oregon. "I believe it is very important for the parents to talk about the birth, whether it was exactly how they planned it or not.

"New parents need someone to tell their story to, and I love to listen," continues Govekar. "It's almost a rite of passage into parenthood. I also use this time to ask their opinion about my care for them before, during, and after the birth. I take all the information they provide me with and use it to better my doula care for future clients."

> "My doula did a postpartum visit two weeks after the birth. It was really nice to talk to her again about the experience and share our perspectives. We looked at pictures from the birth and shared our thoughts. Our talk helped me process and reflect on all that had happened during the birth." —Kari, California

# Doula Dancing

Lying on your back or side may be the most convenient position for your doctor but usually it's the most uncomfortable position to labor in. Your doula can help you find alternative positions and demonstrate movements that can alleviate labor pains and make the contractions more effective.

Here are a few doula dances, as explained to me by Teresa Howard, a doula who has attended over 160 births:

**Walking the halls.** There are several benefits to remaining upright or walking during labor. Physically, your pelvis remains wide and loose, giving the baby room to twist and turn into the proper position for birth. Emotionally, remaining upright can give you a sense of control. "It helps her to not feel like a sick patient and works to help her feel powerful," explains Howard. "In turn, it distracts her from the pain. When she is outside of her room, she has tons to look at and her senses are full . . ."

**Hands and knees.** This position allows the baby the most room to move and is ideal for back labor or any time you'd like to encourage the baby to change positions. "It allows the mom to rest if you put her head on a birth ball and have her hug the ball, not putting any pressure on her hands and stress into her shoulders," explains Howard. "[The doula] has access to her back for massage as well."

**Rocking in a chair or sitting on a birth ball.** These upright positions are more restful than the others. The rocking movement acts as a distraction from the pain. "If she is on a birth ball it is important to have someone either behind her or in front of her at all times," warns Howard. "I prefer to sit her in front of the bed, having pillows to allow her to rest her head on, while I massage her back."

# Doula Dancing (*continued*)

**Back to back with the doula.** In a bed, you and your doula sit back to back. During contractions, your doula pushes against your back, while someone else presses their hands just under your knees. This provides counterpressure. "Putting a heated rice sock or an ice pack between the two backs gives additional help to the mom," advises Howard.

**Half squats, stair climbing, and lunges.** All of these movements may alleviate back labor. These movements open the pelvis, allowing the baby more room to turn.

**Knee press.** The knee press is yet another method of relieving back labor. The doula shapes both hands like the letter V, thumb apart from the rest of her fingers. Then she places each hand at the base of the mother's knees. During a contraction, the doula pushes against the mother's knees, while someone else pushes against the mother's back—or alternatively, while the mother's back is pressing against something hard, like a chair. "It works wonders!" exclaims Howard.

**The Doula Hula.** While standing up, support your upper body by placing your hands onto either a bed raised to the highest position or some other high piece of furniture. Then, move your hips in a belly dance formation. Your husband can stand behind you and support your hips while you sway. "You can turn on some nice music and have [the mother and partner] slow dance as well," says Howard. "Moving the hips helps the mom stay distracted and helps the baby move down at the same time."

# Breastfeeding and the Postpartum Period

I remember my first try at breastfeeding, after my oldest son was born. I was holding the baby, wanting to nurse him. All the breast-feeding books I read said to try nursing the baby right after birth, and I felt like time was running out. But I was nervous. There were people in the room. I wasn't exactly sure how to begin, what I should try, or how I should hold him.

But then a nurse walked in and asked me if I wanted help. She cleared the room. She showed me how to hold him and we tried to get him to latch on. While this attempt didn't get very far, as my baby was sleepy from medication, I truly appreciated the support this nurse gave me. "I loved breastfeeding," she told me, "And I encourage everyone to give it a try. It's hard at first, but it's worth the effort."

If you plan on nursing, your doula can help you with your baby's first meal. She can help you clear the room of family or remind the staff that you'd like to try nursing the baby before they take him away to the nursery or clean him up. While not all doulas are lactation consultants, most have basic knowledge or personal experience with breastfeeding.

"I always like to see the baby nurse once before I leave a new family," explains doula DeeDee Farris-Folkerts. "I find that many times this first nursing is the toughest, and that many problems can be spotted and dealt with right away. If a mom is having problems afterwards, I will come and see if I can help her. I work closely with a La Leche League leader and will call her over if something is outside of my knowledge base or experience. I will also refer to local lactation consultants."

"If I know ahead of time [that my client] will be breastfeeding," says Sue Coffman, a Bradley childbirth educator and doula from California, "then as soon as the mom wants, I help with positioning, skin-to-skin contact, checking baby's latch, and reminding mom she has the ability to do this."

Breastfeeding support goes beyond informational support. Emotional support and encouragement are equally important. Your doula will listen to your worries, answer your "Is this normal?" questions, and be able to refer you to a professional if you're having a problem.

# Extra Comforts

Many doulas provide extra services to their clients. Some are certified childbirth educators and may be able to give you and your partner private lessons. Or she may offer a variety of group classes to her clients.

## CLASSES

"I offer a series of classes called *Developing Trust in Birth*," explains doula DeeDee Farris-Folkerts. "The series was developed for those women who intend to have a drug-free delivery. I have also developed a series of classes for siblings who will be attending the birth of the new baby. I offer this in a very small group setting or one-on-one.

"I also teach prenatal belly dance classes!" says Farris-Folkerts. "The sensual moves

"[My doula] was there when I tried to nurse Nina for the first time. Though her latch was very strong, I couldn't get her latched on properly. Georg'ann, as well as a lactation consultant at the hospital, had great ideas of how to improve her latch and provided a lot of support for what can be a surprisingly difficult technique." —Miriam, Indiana

that we call belly dance were once actually used as a birth dance. When a mother was in labor, other women in the tribe would gather around her and dance. Mimicking birth movements, these women hoped to help the mother have a faster and easier delivery. We now know that being in good physical shape helps tremendously during childbearing. The mother will stretch, tone, learn to move her pelvis freely, gain control over her abdominal muscles, and have a great time!"

## GIFTS

Your doula may give you a book or other small gift. Some doulas give their clients a birth ball, or they give the mother a homemade rice sock. A rice sock is a pouch, sometimes a sock sewn closed, filled with rice that you warm up in the microwave and place against the body, providing pain relief.

"I knit booties for all my clients," says doula Elizabeth Lott. "I am usually behind on bootie production, so I often end up giving clients the very booties I was working on as I waited for their 'We're going to the hospital now' call."

> [My doula] gave us a written account of the labor and birth. I thought it'd be clinically written, but instead it was one of the most poetic and moving pieces of prose I've ever read. I keep those pages in a safe place, and whenever I read it, I'm moved to tears." —Yonit, Indiana

## DOCUMENTATION

"I do birth stories for every family," says doula Cyndi Whitwell. "So I am taking notes during the labor, finishing them up after the baby is out, and then typing them up, about a week after the postpartum visit. This gives them clear details of the timing of the labor for them to tell their terrific birth story to others.

"I also take disposable cameras on every birth," continues Whitwell. "If they don't have anyone specifically involved in taking pictures, I do it during labor and right after the birth (dad cutting

# Recording the Birth

Weddings, anniversaries, graduations, the baby's first steps. We use pictures and video to capture moments like these in our lives. Why not take pictures or video at the birth of your child?

"I tell people that if they are wishy-washy about it at all, to do it, because you can destroy tapes and photos, but you can't go back and take them if you decide later you want them," says Stephanie Soderblom, doula and owner of *BirthDiaries.com*. "I tell them that rarely do people even know that photos are being taken. Often the video camera is turned on and placed on a tripod or on a table and left, and I don't use a flash, so it's not intrusive."

Here are some tips on recording the birth of your child:

* First, check with your doctor or midwife and the hospital or birth center where you will be delivering. Some doctors will not allow video to be taken during the actual birth, but before and after is okay. Some hospitals do not allow any video, but they do allow still photographs. Or you may need to sign papers stating that you'll turn the camera off if asked.

* Be prepared. Bring two cameras, extra film, and extra batteries. If you're videotaping the birth, bring two empty tapes, and record on extended play.

* Consider taking photos in black-and-white instead of color. Black-and-white photos soften the birth colors.

* Designate your doula or a family member to take the pictures. Or you can hire someone. Just be sure to decide before labor begins. Ask the photographer to remain "invisible." In other words, ask them not to disrupt the birth by asking you to smile or pose, and make sure they stay out of the caregiver's way.

## Recording the Birth (*continued*)

* "Rather than taking a photo because you can, I try to capture a moment," advises Soderblom. "A closeup of the brand-new baby holding daddy's finger, the look of the baby's face as it's being born, the look on mom's face as she meets her baby for the first time. When taping video, I will often set the scene. If it's snowing outside, I'll begin with a view through the hospital window at the snowy trees, then zoom out and pan over to see mom in labor."

* You don't have to take pictures of the actual birth. Modest pictures can be taken, or you can limit photos to before real labor begins and after the baby is born. Just be sure the camera or camcorder is nearby, and your doula or designated photographer knows she should start taking pictures as soon as the baby has arrived.

cord, mom holding baby, etc.). Then I give them the camera. They have the control to throw it away or develop as they please."

Some doulas create birth art with their clients, like belly casts or painting symbolic pictures of pregnancy and childbirth.

"I offer belly casts," says Farris-Folkerts. "I lube mom's breasts, belly and arms with KY or Vaseline and then lay strips of gauze with plaster casting over her. Once I am finished and we give it a few minutes to cure, we carefully remove the cast and let it sit for 24 hours. Then it is sanded and I apply several coats of a white sealant called Gesso. This is a several-day process. Then it is done and ready for decoration! Moms love having this 3-D piece of art to commemorate their beautiful pregnant selves!"

CHAPTER 4

# Dads and Doulas

UNTIL RECENTLY, FATHERS WERE not deeply involved with the pregnancy, let alone the birth, of their child. When birth was at home, the mother was supported by her midwife and other female relatives or friends, and when women began laboring in hospitals, the father was not permitted into the labor or delivery room. This is where the image of a father pacing the halls of a hospital, waiting to hear if he's the proud new father of a boy or girl, originated.

In the late 1960s, women demanded that fathers play a more active role in the parenting scene, including childbirth. Hospitals reluctantly allowed fathers to attend. Today, fathers are not only welcome but encouraged to attend the birth, and many hospitals allow fathers to attend c-section births as well.

While obviously fathers should be permitted to attend the birth of their child, and it's wonderful that they are playing a more active role, a question remains unanswered: What role should the father take during labor and childbirth?

> ## 🐾 A BIRTHING MOMENT . . .
>
> "After our baby was first delivered and they took her to the side to do all the tests and get her cleaned up, I was torn at first because I knew my wife still had to deliver the afterbirth. But I did want to go see our precious baby. That was when the doula said that it was okay for me to go and that she would stay with my wife and make sure she was okay. With a nod from my wife, I went to the side and adored our daughter. It was at that point that I was really grateful for the doula and all she had done for us." —William, Florida

# Dad's Role

Childbirth education classes attempt to include the father in the birth by assigning him the role of "birth coach." He's encouraged to take charge and, if they are trying for an unmedicated birth, help his wife cope without drugs. But what if the wife "loses control," as many women do during birth? What if the mother does need medication? Or what if the father feels overwhelmed seeing his wife in pain and cannot remember what he was taught in class? Then the father may feel he has failed in his role.

Fathers should not be forced into a position that they are not properly prepared for or may not be emotionally capable of. Yes, fathers should be at the birth of their child, if they feel comfortable being there. But they should be free to act as fathers, not forced into the role of birth coaches. They should not feel pressured to relieve their wives of pain or need to remember the details of their birth plans. They should be free to worry, cry, and experience the birth of their child and themselves as a new father.

This is not to say that fathers can't make great birth coaches! Some fathers are wonderful birth coaches. They study the birth books, take childbirth education classes seriously, and practice with the mother at home. Then at the birth they support their wives, remember everything they learned in class, and experience the occasion without feeling pressured and overly anxious. But this is the exception.

Of course, mothers still need support in labor, and this support can come from the doula.

# How Doulas Support Dads

Doulas aren't just there for mom; they help fathers as well. How do doulas help dads?

- *Guilt-free breaks.* Labor typically lasts 8 to 15 hours, depending on a variety of factors. It may last longer than 20 hours! A doula can remind dad to take breaks, get something to eat, or even take a nap. He won't have to worry about leaving his wife alone, as the doula will be right by her side. Frank, a new father, says, "The most tangible help was that she and I acted as a kind of 'tag-team' birth partner. For example, she would massage Christine's back or spray hot water on her belly (in the birthing tub), or she would spell me for a while if I needed to just sit and close my eyes—we labored all night. Or she would run and get drinks or snacks. She essentially was my right-hand person during the labor. I know that the primary role of the doula is to comfort the mother, but fathers and birth partners need to realize that since the partner's primary role is also to aid and comfort the birthing mother, the doula will be an enormous help and support to them."

## 🐦 A BIRTHING MOMENT . . .

"My doulas poured water over my back when it felt good, and they stopped as soon as I snapped that it wasn't working anymore. They immediately noticed that I didn't have anything to drink and went to get some water for me. They warmed up my rice sock and brought me cool cloths for my head. They also videotaped and photographed my birth, and that was something I really wanted. But I think the most important thing was to let me and my husband be together. In my other two labors, my husband had seemed very distant, and I was very afraid that if I seemed weak, it would only drive him further away. This labor went so much faster, and the baby was [sunny side up], so I was really in a lot more pain. I couldn't think about how my actions would affect my husband. I could only labor. I held on to my husband for most of my labor, and he was right there for me. And so even though it was physically my hardest labor, it was also my best labor." —Lucky, Wisconsin

- *Helping dads be helpful.* Sometimes dad wants to help, but he's not sure where to begin. Or he may feel intimidated by the medical staff coming in and out of the room. The doula can empower him to support his wife.
- *Emotional support.* Mothers aren't the only ones riding an emotional roller coaster: Dads have feelings too! They may go from excited, to nervous, to worried, to confused, to joyful and relieved. When an emergency or unusual situation arises, the father may be left on the sidelines with little or no explanation from the medical staff as they attend to his wife

"I attended a birth where the mom had an epidural, and when it came time to push, she had a very specific idea of what she wanted. She asked dad to sit in the bed behind her, but he was surprised and very reluctant. I encouraged him to try, and told him that if it really didn't work, he could change positions. He took off his shoes, climbed in the bed behind her, and held her as she pushed. He whispered in her ear, supported her as she curled around the baby to push, and later said he felt like he was giving birth with her. He also told me how much it had meant to him that I had encouraged him to at least try, because he might have missed out on such a special role if I had not been encouraging about it." —Ana M. Hill, CLD CD, Colorado

and unborn child. A doula can make sure he understands what the situation is, if there really is something to worry about, or if all is going well.

- *Less pressure.* With a doula present, the couple will not need to worry about forgetting their birth plans or trying to remember the pros and cons of interventions. Also, for a father who wishes to take a backseat, a doula allows him to relax and experience the birth without being actively involved. One father greatly appreciated that a doula was there to comfort his wife and help her cope. He says, "I am not good at that kind of thing, and it wouldn't have been natural for me to calm her very well. The doula took the active role, and I observed. I appreciated that."

# Commonly Asked Questions

While doulas seem to be the best choice for the mother, most dads-to-be have a few concerns. Here are the three most commonly asked questions

Q. **"I want the birth to be a private event, between my wife and myself. I don't think I'll feel comfortable with a stranger in the room. Won't the doula's presence ruin the intimacy of the birth?"**

A. If you equate intimacy with being alone, then you're in for a big surprise! It's normal to have anywhere from three to six people in the room at a hospital birth. People walk in and out without knocking, and you will have never met most of the staff. On the other hand, you will have met with your doula at least once, if not more times, before delivery.

According to the research, a doula's presence may actually improve your relationship. One study asked mothers to compare their

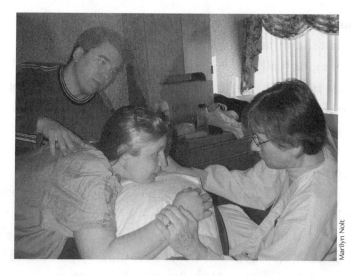

FIGURE 4.1.  Dads and doulas work together
to provide perfect support.

"There is no such thing as privacy in a hospital, even in the birthing ward, and you just have to expect that you will not be alone for more than two minutes. (You might be, but you can't count on it.) The doulas were very good about stepping out from time to time (either at my request or of their own choice) to give us some time alone. They would even stand guard at the door and ask the nurse to come back in a few minutes! They were not strangers; they were part of the experience." —Dan, Colorado

relationship with their partners before and after the baby's birth. Seventy percent of the mothers who had a doula reported feeling more satisfied with their relationship at six weeks postpartum. Only 30 percent of the moms who did not have a doula felt their relationship improved after the birth. (Klaus & Kennell, 1997)

"I strongly believe that it is a doula's job to support and enhance a relationship between the mom and dad and not to interfere with the intimate nature of their relationship," explains certified doula and childbirth educator Kathryn Berkowitz. "The memories that a mother has of her husband quietly stroking her hair or rubbing her back or showing her compassion during labor and birth is something that many women will treasure for a lifetime. These things go a long way into building strong marriages and lifelong commitments. Birth is an intimate family event, and I am an honored guest who believes in protecting the sacredness of that moment."

Q. "We attended childbirth education classes. They taught me how to support my wife and told us what to expect. What can the doula tell us or help us with that we can't do ourselves?"

"Unless you deliver babies for a living, you don't have the experience. I'll give this male response, since I used this for a friend. Would you prefer to have someone fix the brakes in your car after he's only had an all-day weekend course and read a book, or would your prefer someone who's changed brakes many times before in a variety of different situations, on different makes and models of cars? Also, a childbirth class will never adequately prepare you for all aspects of childbirth. Our doula brought a number of relaxation items that helped, and we hadn't seriously considered some of them."
—Don, California

$A.$ There is a big difference between reading about childbirth or watching videos of others in labor and actually supporting a woman in labor or seeing your wife give birth. The classes are great for lessening the fear of the unknown and presenting your options, but when it comes to labor support, hands-on experience is extremely helpful.

A doula has not only received specialized training but has also attended other births. Plus, she's used to seeing women labor. You may feel upset or nervous, worrying that something is wrong. It's difficult to remember what you learned in class when emotions are running high. Your doula, on the other hand, is comfortable with the ways of birth and will remain objective.

"It is an injustice to send partners through a class and then tell them they can handle labor with what they have been taught," says LaNette J. McQuitty, a certified doula and childbirth educator in Wisconsin. "We should tell partners that they possess the power to comfort deep within, and what we teach is to not learn a way, but to feel a way, to ease the journey."

Q. **"If the doula will be supporting my wife, then what will I have to do?"**

A. Doulas do not replace fathers. As my doula, Dianne Lentine, told my husband, "I won't be there telling her how much I love her. That's your job." Doulas provide practical support, but fathers radiate strength and love to their partners.

For dads who want to be actively involved in the birth, a doula can guide him on how to support his wife. The combination of the doula's knowledge and experience with the father's loving touch or voice can make all the difference in the world—less stress on the father, and perfect loving support for the mother.

"I tell my clients during our prenatal visit that ten, twenty, or fifty years later, when my name has been long forgotten, she will still remember everything that her partner said and did during her labor," explains tracy hartley, certified doula from California. "My job is to make him look good in that memory."

> "I felt as if having a doula might diminish my role to the point where I wasn't even needed. But after meeting with our doula, I felt much better, and my trepidation about having her there was gone. Helen, our doula, kept me involved with the birth, and it was nice to feel like I didn't have to know everything." —Ben, Ohio

# When Dad Is Unsure

Sometimes, mom wants a doula, but dad is not sure. He's nervous. Worried that the doula will take away his role, concerned that the doula won't be worth the money, or pondering similar questions that we've reviewed in this chapter.

I asked some fathers the following question: If your friend told you his wife wanted a doula, but he wasn't sure if he wanted a doula, what would you tell him? Here are some of their answers:

- *Billy:* I would probably share how wonderful and fulfilling it made our second child's birthing experience, especially after our first was not what we wanted, but we were hesitant to speak up. She provides a lot of confidence, calming you and your wife, and spreads out the labor experience between more than just you and your wife.

- *Mark:* I would advise him to really consider getting the doula. It is his wife having the baby after all and the doulas do a lot to help them deal with labor in their own way and that alone takes part of the burden off the husband. When you think about all the money you'll spend on your baby in the first year, the cost of a doula is really inconsequential."

- *Nick:* "Here's a question: would you go to court to argue your own case in a lawsuit? I imagine most people would want an attorney present—somebody who can guide and advise you through a stressful and unfamiliar event. A doula plays a similar role for an expecting couple. Keep in mind that during childbirth, nobody but a doula will be there to advocate on your behalf. The doctor or midwife will show up minutes before the actual birth, and they have their own agenda. You are completely overwhelmed and caught up in the situation. The doula is the only person who can keep a level head and be completely on your side."

## CHAPTER 5

# Doulas and Epidurals

A POPULAR PARENTING MAGAZINE published a feature story on doulas and epidurals. The article, which was solely based on the negative experience of the author, warned women not to hire a doula unless they're die-hard "natural childbirth" fans. Unfortunately, this article fed into a common myth that doulas are only for women who are attempting to give birth without drugs or medical intervention. Nothing could be further from the truth.

Doulas are there to provide emotional, informational, and physical support. Women who receive medication during labor need all of the above, and in some situations, even more so than women who choose to avoid medication. Let's take a closer look at some of the myths surrounding doulas and epidurals, and then examine exactly how doulas serve mothers who choose, or require, medication for labor and childbirth.

## Myth Versus Fact

*Myth:* **Doulas are only interested in supporting women who plan on giving birth without medication.**

🍃  A BIRTHING MOMENT . . .

"I successfully labored at home, walking and taking hot showers. My doula suggested ways to get rest between contractions, which seemed less than regular. She suggested different positions for laboring but encouraged me to do what seemed most natural for me, which was walking. She encouraged me to snack on light foods and drink to keep my strength up. She helped me labor at home until my water broke, and then protocol dictated our arrival at the hospital. That was one of my main objectives—to labor at home as long as possible, and I know for a fact that we would have ended up at the hospital so much sooner, only to be strapped to a bed.

Upon arrival at the hospital, we discovered that both my doctor and the anesthesiologist were in surgery, and I had to wait for my epidural. My doula helped me cope somewhat with the strong contractions. I felt like I was losing control, and she continued to remind me that I was doing a great job and following the needs of my body. What a comforting presence my doula provided!" —Denise, Maryland

*Fact:* Doulas want every woman to have a positive and empowering birth experience. For some women, that means giving birth with as little intervention as possible. For others, laboring without medication is not even a consideration, either for personal or practical reasons.

From the personal side, many mothers are afraid of the unknown. What if the pain gets worse? Will I be able to cope? What if I wait too long and then they won't give me any medication? What will it feel like when the head is being born? What if I need an emergency c-section? With all these thoughts flying around, it's extremely difficult to relax and let birth happen, and fear intensifies pain. Ob-

"My doula helped me to achieve what I wanted from birth. I wanted to labor without meds, although my doctor required an epidural for the birth [because I was expecting twins]. I knew if I labored with meds, I'd be confined to bed and that is not what I wanted.... [My doula] and I discussed options, and we decided to approach my doctor with this solution: have the anesthesiologist put the epidural catheter in my back in early labor, but not run any meds until I asked. My doctor thought this would work. In actuality, I did labor without any meds—to 10 centimeters." —Lori, Wisconsin

viously, a fearful birth is the opposite of a positive and empowering one, and no doula wants her client to experience birth as a traumatic event.

There are insistences when medication is required for labor. While a doula is trained to view birth as a natural and normal process, she's aware that there is a time and place for medical intervention.

*Myth:* **Doulas push their opinions and philosophies onto their clients.**

*Fact:* Doulas provide their clients with information so they can make informed decisions. Then the doula's job is to support the choices. A doula does not make decisions for a couple, and she should not provide biased information.

"I am constantly educating from the day I am hired," explains Wendy Spry, a certified doula in California. "In the heat of the moment, I go back to the birth plan they wrote and reiterate the benefits and risks of the choices they are going to make. I make sure we have time alone without staff present and give a chance for clear heads to prevail. When the decision is made, I support it with all that I have. I feel a personal obligation to be sure they know all benefits and risks before making any decision. I would hate for the couple to come back to me after the fact and say, 'Why didn't you tell me?' They can only make an informed and empowering decision if they have all the facts."

*Myth:* **A doula will make me feel guilty if I "chicken out" and choose to use medication.**

"I interviewed my doula and asked her point-blank, 'What if I decide I want to have an epidural or other medication? Will you be okay with that?' The last thing I need at a time of great stress is to worry about someone else's political views of birth. She was very open [to me receiving medication during labor]."
—Amy, Texas

*Fact:* Your doula will support you and your choices. Your doula is not interested in making martyrs out of her clients. She is interested in helping women have the best birth experience possible, with the healthiest outcome.

"[For women who want to try having a non-medicated birth,] I tell her that I like to use what I call a rule of three," explains Kathy Clark, a doula from Colorado. "She asks for pain medication three times in a row, and then I know she is serious and wants the medication.... If she thinks that is a good way to do it, that's what we do. If she wants it to be only one time, I tell her that I will repeat to her what she had 'planned' prenatally and see if she has changed her mind, or is just looking for reassurance that this is normal and that she is doing a good job. I tell her I will not lie to her. That if she isn't coping well, I will be honest with her. Most important, I want her to understand that the true definition of a doula is women helping women, not women making decisions or judgments for other women."

### 🐾 A BIRTHING MOMENT . . .

"I remember telling my doula that I thought I needed to go to the bathroom and it felt like a bowel movement. I couldn't imagine this to be true, and how I would manage since I had an epidural and couldn't walk to the toilet! But Peggy patiently told me she was pretty sure it was the pressure of the baby. Sure enough, the labor nurse checked, and I was a full 10 centimeters! If I had been alone at that time, I would've freaked out thinking I would have to deal with going to the bathroom and how I would manage to get out of bed!"
—Rebecca, Washington

*Myth:* **Women who use medication during childbirth do not need the services of a professional labor support person. There will be nothing for the doula to do.**

*Fact:* Women who plan on using medication for labor pains still go through the emotional roller coaster ride of childbirth, and they still need to make informed decisions regarding interventions. Women who plan on using medication are not "pain free," and they may need more help than nonmedicated mothers during the pushing stages. In short, epidurals do not replace doulas.

"Epidurals and other medications do not remind the family members to eat," explains Tabitha Trotter, a certified doula in California. "They do not remind mom to roll over, they do not fetch extra pillows. I feel a doula is needed for every birth, including cesarean! The doula can help take care of other family members ('Now's a good time to go get something to eat.' 'You should probably try to take a nap while mom's resting.'), and continue to be a resource for mom and the family if complications arise. The reassurance a doula brings is needed by all."

# Medicated Labor

With the exception of an induction or c-section, no one starts labor medicated, and many doctors require women to be 4 or 5 centimeters dilated before receiving an epidural. Plus, with so many women requesting medication for labor, you may wait an hour or longer before getting the epidural. A doula can help you cope with labor pains until you receive medicated pain relief.

> "My doula supported my decision for an epidural after she and my husband made sure that it was truly what I wanted. When it took the anesthesiologist an hour and a half to show up, my doula was the one who helped me through the pain. She also convinced the nurse to turn down the Pitocin until I got the epidural." —Peri, Florida

## EPIDURALS

While receiving an epidural, your doula can help you remain still and cope with any contractions that may come. If you'd like your husband to hold you, the doula can tell him how to hold you, and then provide any emotional support you need, either by holding your hand or offering words of reassurance.

Epidurals do not always provide complete relief from pain. Sometimes the mother can still feel pain on one side of her body, or in a certain area. Depending on the length of labor, the epidural may wear off and need to be refilled. Unlike a mother who gives birth without medication and has time to get used to each contraction as they grow stronger, if your epidural wears off, you may become suddenly overwhelmed and feel panicked when you go from no pain to transitional contractions. Your doula will help you cope with the sudden pain.

# Finding a Doula for a Medicated Birth

It would be dishonest for me to tell you that every doula supports women who want a medicated childbirth. The majority of doulas, however, support mothers who plan on using an epidural or narcotics, and a few even specialize in medicated birth empowerment. How do you find a doula that will honestly support your choices?

While we will talk more about hiring a doula in chapter 7, here are some tips on hiring a doula for a medicated labor:

- Before you mention that you're planning on using medication, ask the doula what her philosophies are regarding childbirth. Ask her how she feels about natural childbirth, and then ask her what she thinks about medicated childbirth. Don't just pay attention to the doula's answers, but also listen to her tone of voice when referring to the use of medication during birth.

- Ask the doula for some real-life examples of how she supported women who chose medication for labor. If your doula says she's never attended a birth where the woman needed medication, unless she is a new doula, take this as a red flag. This may not be the right doula for your birth.

- Watch out for doulas who advertise that they've never had a mother need medication. The doula may eager to keep her "good record," and besides, if she's never attended a mother who has used an epidural, she may not know how to support you as well as a doula who has.

"Medication is not a substitute for support," explains Devorah Shulman, a doula from New York. "Even though the pain is no longer something they have to deal with to the same extent, there is still fear. Women still need reassurance. They still need their ice chips. They still get hot and sweaty. They still might need massage. In many medicated births, the sensation of pain increases as the baby descends through the pelvis and second stage approaches. Someone who's not expecting to feel any pain whatsoever needs support."

On the other hand, your epidural may work too well. During the pushing stages, being able to feel the baby and work with the contractions is practically impossible when you're numb from the waist down. Some doctors will "turn the epidural down" so you can feel just enough to push effectively, but from personal experience, I can tell you this really does not help. Your doula can coach you on how and when to push. She will also help support you in whatever position you're pushing in.

> "I had an epidural, and during the actual birth, our doula took pictures so that my husband could participate in the birth, and after the birth, she assisted me with a first feeding. There were definite roles that I wanted my doula to fill that had nothing to do with having an epidural." —Sara, Texas

## NARCOTICS

Epidurals are not the only medications used to help moms cope with pain. Narcotics do not provide pain relief, but attempt to relax the mother so she can rest in between contractions. Narcotics make some women feel worse. They may become nauseous or disoriented, feel confused, or unable to focus and work with their bodies when contractions come. A doula will stay nearby and hold your hand if you're feeling lost or scared, clean up vomit, wipe a cool cloth on

### 🐦 A BIRTHING MOMENT . . .

"For the twin birth, I labored standing for the most part. I alternated between leaning forward with my upper body on the bed, but standing. I sat intermittently. I began to have the terrible pains I had with my first birth—pains radiating from my hips all the way up my back. At this point, Annmarie placed her hands on my hips and applied pressure with every contraction. The pain was gone.

"The nurses walked in on my laboring—standing bent over the bed, with Annmarie applying pressure to my hips. I was very in control, 'in the zone' so to speak. I was not in pain, but making very loud birthing sounds. The moaning helped me release the pain vocally. When one nurse said to the other, 'Now there is a mom who knows how to labor!' I was never so proud in my life." —Lori, Washington

your head, or get a nurse if you need her.

After an epidural is in place, you'll be unable to get up or walk around. Your doula can get whatever you need, whether it is ice chips or a cool cloth. If your partner is exhausted and wants to rest, or he'd like to get something to eat, your doula will be there so you won't feel alone. She may give you a massage or make sure you have enough pillows and are comfortable. She'll be there if you want to talk. Or

"Once the epidural is administered, you still have to push and you still have to breathe. Because you are not feeling the contractions, it almost makes the role of the doula more significant—in fact, I would say it does make her role more significant. She is your signal for breathing. She is your signal for pushing." —Sara, Texas

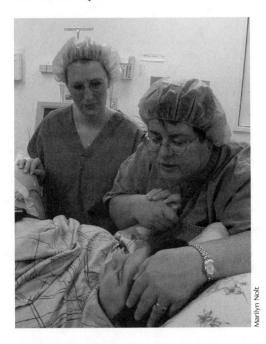

FIGURE 5.1. As mom is prepared for surgery, her doula remains nearby.

Marilyn Nolt

"Just because you have pain medication, you aren't immune to the effects of labor. I ended up with an epidural after a horrible labor brought on by inducing drugs. Once the epidural was in place, labor became manageable. But it wasn't pain-free; I still was completely taken by each contraction that occurred after the epidural. Peggy maintained my focus throughout."
—Rebecca, Washington

she may play checkers or card games with you! Whatever you want, whatever you need, she is there for you.

## OTHER INTERVENTIONS

Unfortunately, once medication is used during birth, other interventions tend to follow. A doula can help the family understand the pros and cons of any additional interventions. Informational support is extremely important for a mom who chooses medication. After a mother already has an IV or is already receiving medication, care providers tend to stop asking the mother if a particular intervention is okay, and just do it. A doula can help remind the couple that they still have choices, and she can encourage them to ask questions and be active participants in their baby's birth.

Emotional support is a vital aspect of doula care during a medicated birth. Fear of what may happen next, guilt over using medication (even when that was planned previously), or the normal mix of excitement and concern that a new mom-to-be experiences as she prepares to become a mother—all of these emotions are difficult to process on your own, and your partner may not be able to relate or understand. Your doula will listen and try to answer your questions and concerns, or she will make sure they are answered by someone knowledgeable.

"She made my husband part of my birth. She relaxed him, calmed his fears, explained things step by step, gave him the chance to take a break out of the room when he needed to, told him the things that would most likely annoy a laboring mom! (I would pay millions for this service; my husband is the authority on annoyance when I am in pain!)." —Jamie, Florida

"[The mother] may need a lot of reassurance that she made the right decision," explains Kathy Clark, a doula and nurse in Colorado. "I think that women who have medicated labors tend to receive less personal care from health providers, and therefore I believe it follows that they receive less information. I think because they are drugged that the staff may feel there is no need to 'bother the mom.' Depending on the type of medication they choose, they may be tied down with every type of corded intervention made.

"If the choice is [narcotic pain relief]," Clark continues, "the mom loses her sense of time, what has occurred, who is there or why, and so they need someone there just touching them all the time

### 🐾 A BIRTHING MOMENT . . .

"I was induced, which alone can be a scary and traumatic experience. I pushed for 3½ hours, and several times they said the words
*vacuum* and *forceps*, but [my doula] encouraged me that I could do
it. I found out later that they were prepping the surgical room for
an emergency c-section, which, had it taken another 15 minutes,
might have been necessary. With her encouragement, plus fantastic
nurses, I did end up delivering without any of those. But at the end
things got hairy, the fetal heartbeat dropped, I had to push when
there was no contraction, and they said they had to cut me because the baby needed to come out now. So they literally ripped
the baby from me and ran her to the neo-care area. Everything was
a daze: where was my baby, did my husband cut the cord, what is
going on? But [my doula] was sitting by me and reassuring me
when no one else could; at that moment, all focus went to my limp
newborn. Except [my doula's] focus, she held my hand and reassured me. My husband was so split in where he should be, and he
was definitely worried, I could see it in every muscle of his body
and face. But not Judy, she sat next to me and focused on me and
no one else. She sat there [for 45 minutes] as they stitched my
fourth-degree episiotomy and waited until finally, an hour later,
they laid a very big and pink baby on my stomach." —Elspeth,
North Carolina

to take away the sensation of being in this all alone. I always hold my
client's hand when she sleeps, so that if she begins to wake, I can talk
in a soothing voice, telling her how well things are going, who all is
there, helping her change positions, and if they want to do a proce-

dure, making sure that she has knowledge of the plan before it is done. And after the baby is born, I help her get her baby ASAP. Medicated moms need less physical support than one who is not [using medication], but they clearly need the comforting, verbal, and emotional support. And someone watching over them."

## CHAPTER 6

# Your Support Team

A DOULA IS ONLY one member of your labor and delivery support team. Depending on where you deliver, members may include nurses, doctors, midwives, midwife assistants, anesthesiologists, and others. Every member has different priorities, training, and goals. Understanding what the key players' roles are and how they interact with your doula will help you have a peaceful birth environment.

## Nurses

With the exception of your doula, your nurse will have the most contact with you during labor and delivery. Your nurse is responsible for attending to your basic medical needs, checking vital signs, answering questions, monitoring and adjusting equipment, administering medications, placing IVs, taking blood, charting your labor and birth, and reporting to the doctor. She may be responsible for more than four patients, or if you're lucky and you go into labor on a good day, you may be one of two.

Often the nurse will carry out orders for your doctor without you ever speaking to the doctor in person. She often acts as the go-between

### ❧ A BIRTHING MOMENT...

"My doula immediately established a comfortable [relationship] with the hospital staff and was great about chatting with the nurse. She would tell [the nurse] that I was doing good, that I was comfortable, etcetera. I hardly had to interact with anyone until it was time to push. The nurse even agreed to let me stay on my birth ball to monitor Caleb's heartbeat, and just checked it for a couple of minutes instead of the usual 20 minutes. She only monitored me twice during labor, and no one checked my dilation until it was time to push—and that was because I asked! I really believe that Terri's presence and obvious competency made them feel better about leaving me to myself, and that the privacy and peace helped my labor progress quickly." —Paula, Georgia

and is there to get what you need from the medical staff. For example, if you want medication, your nurse will be the one to contact your doctor and ask him under what circumstances it is it acceptable for you to have medication. She may contact a resident or wait for your doctor to check cervical dilation, then find the anesthesiologist and place an IV if one is not already in place. Nurses will update your chart and tend to a variety of other tasks. Needless to say, your nurse will be very busy, especially if the hospital is understaffed.

Many nurses become labor and delivery nurses because they want to support women in labor, but practically speaking, they cannot be with one patient continuously. Even if there is a one-to-one ratio between nurses and patients, the nurse is still responsible for performing medical tasks, charting, and carrying out doctor's orders. A doula has only one responsibility—to provide continuous emotional and physical support for you. The roles of the nurse and doula do not overlap but actually complement each other.

"One nurse told me that I did all the things she wished she had the time to do," says Emily Murray, a certified doula in Maine. "I think she felt a lot of pressure was taken off her shoulders knowing that the couple's emotional needs were being taken care of. She would come in to check on the progress, offer wise and wonderful advice, and then leave to check on her other patients without feeling like the couple was being neglected."

Many nurses welcome doulas, while others are apprehensive. "The issues arise when doulas are thrust into a hospital setting where their role is not well defined for the nursing staff," explains Shirley Picard, a nurse manager at Memorial Hospital in Rhode Island and certified labor doula. "Some nurses may have had experiences with doulas who have stepped outside of their scope of practice; in other words, performing nursing tasks, offering medical advice, or contradicting care providers.

"Other reservations with doulas stem from some feelings

> "Many requests were made with a please and thank you for blankets, drinks, or directions. I felt no tension among my birth team. My doulas were very respectful of the nurses and the midwife for the space they needed for my birth. . . . When there is trust and respect among all parties about what each can and can't do, there is an invaluable amount of cooperation and feeling of flow that can be achieved." —Kelley, North Carolina

that the doula may take over the best part of their job," Picard continues. "The reality is that there's more than enough work to do in supporting a woman through birth. When doulas and nurses share this task, it creates a positive atmosphere whereby the nurse can

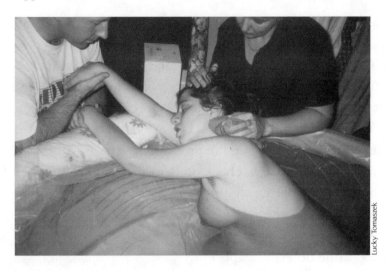

FIGURE 6.1. Homebirth is a safe alternative for women with normal pregnancies. In the comfort of her home, this mom receives strength from her husband, while her doula gently pats her neck with a cool cloth.

attend to other requirements of her job, like documentation and other assigned patients."

If a nurse is overwhelmingly negative about your doula's presence, or if she is in any other way intimidating or making your birth atmosphere tense, you have a right to ask for another nurse. It's best to have either you or your partner request the new nurse. If the doula were to ask for a new nurse, it may only strengthen the nurse's negativity. Of course, if you feel intimidated and the doula is the only person present to make the request besides yourself, then do not hesitate to ask for your doula's help.

# Doctors

Obstetricians are responsible for prenatal care, treating any complications that arise, and labor and delivery care. By nature, obstetricians maintain a medical view of pregnancy and labor with the emphasis of their training on high-risk and unusual situations. While the doctor attends to the mother's medical needs, the doula attends to the mother's emotional and practical needs.

At one of your prenatal appointments, you'll want to mention to your doctor that you plan on having a doula present for the birth. If he seems positive about the idea, then great! If he seems negative or apprehensive, he may not understand the true role of the doula, or he may have had a bad experience with an unprofessional doula. It may help if you explain that the doula is there for your emotional well-being and to provide labor support, and you trust the doctor to provide medical advice and services. Ask your doula if she'd be willing to attend one of your prenatal appointments. At this appointment, the doula can address any concerns or answer questions regarding the doula's role.

If your doctor still seems negative, you have a choice. Assuming you want a doula, you can either ignore the doctor's negativity, hoping your birth and doula will serve as a good example, or you can switch doctors. You do not want anyone at the birth, especially your key care provider, feeling apprehensive or upset with your choices of labor companions. It's your decision ultimately, and you should not feel intimidated to choose your doula over your doctor or vice versa.

If you receive care from a group of doctors, you'll want to mention your desire for doula support to each member of the group. Your favorite doctor in the group may love doulas, but if one of his partners has a negative attitude, and he's on-call the night you go into labor, you may find yourself in a tense situation!

When you go into labor, depending on the hospital and your doctor's policies, you will be examined by either a resident or your own doctor. Your doctor will determine whether he considers you to be in active labor. Depending on your current situation and your doctor's philosophy of birth, the doctor may suggest an intervention or medication or may suggest nothing and allow labor to continue normally. If an intervention is suggested, your doula may be able to explain the pros and cons of the intervention, or she may encourage you to ask the doctor to explain why he feels this intervention is necessary. It is up to you and your partner, however, to decide if this is something you'd like to do or if you'd rather take a "wait and see" approach.

## DOULA AND DOCTOR: ONE WOMAN'S STORY

Doula Shirley M. Picard, of Rhode Island, tells of a positive experience with a physician:

"[I was working as a doula for] a woman who was laboring with her third baby, and she had had two previous vaginal deliveries. The baby had a prolonged fetal heart rate deceleration, and we transferred the woman to the operating room for an emergency cesarean section. Thankfully, by the time we got everything set up in the operating room, the fetal heart rate had recovered to its baseline. This normally impatient, high-intervention obstetrician sat it out and then asked us to take her back to the labor room to see if she could deliver vaginally. The obstetrician told us that this patient's baby was in a direct occiput posterior position, and he thought that she would probably end up sectioned anyway.

"With that, the other nurse and I got an idea. We asked him to give us 20 minutes without any interference from him. We were going to try something, but he needed to trust us, and stay out of the room. This was a man of few words, who had a reputation for intimidating the nursing staff. He said, 'Do whatever. I'll be back in 20 minutes.'

"We got this woman up on the side of the bed and had her lunging back and forth. At 18½ minutes, in walks the obstetrician (he just couldn't wait the full 20!), just as we see this baby rotate and rapidly descend. He never had enough time to gown and glove. I ended up delivering the head. Afterwards, he said, 'Thank you, good job,' smiled and left. The nurse and I were just delighted it had worked!

"A week or so later, I get a knock on my office door (I am also a nurse manager here.) It's the same doctor saying, 'I need you now. Come do that thing you do.' Same scenario as before, without the operating room run, but an occiput posterior baby, wedged in tight.

Again, lunging was successful, and this time he didn't leave the room—just watched. After the delivery, he said, 'It's about time the nurses start paying attention to the patients and not the monitors and machines. You are doing a good job!' We all sat there in disbelief as we realized that the biggest doctor challenge we had was now our biggest supporter! He has been awesome, open to suggestions and questions —and always giving us the benefit of the doubt."

Sometimes, doctors and doulas collide on this issue. Some may feel that the doula is questioning the doctor's suggestion by encouraging you to ask questions before approving an act. When in actuality, the doula is simply encouraging the expectant mother to give informed consent. This protects both the mother, in that she understands why and what they are doing, and the doctor, who then knows that his patient understands his approach to the situation.

There are several "right answers" when it comes to managing labor. Breaking a woman's bag of waters, for example, is performed routinely by some doctors, while others would never consider the idea unless something is wrong. It's your responsibility to find out if the intervention they wish to perform is routine or if it is necessary. If it is simply routine, your doula can help you understand the pros and cons so you can make an informed choice. An honest doula and doctor will not imply that there is a correct answer to these types of questions, but instead, the doctor and doula should work together to help you decide what risks you would or would not like to take. If you decide in favor of the intervention, the doctor will carry out the intervention or prescribe orders, while your doula will support your choice and explain what you should expect to happen during or after the intervention is carried out.

# Midwives

Midwives and doulas are often thought to be of the same profession, but this is untrue. Midwives, like obstetricians, provide prenatal care

## ❧ A BIRTHING MOMENT . . .

"My husband and son and I went out to breakfast, to take my mind off what I thought was early labor, but I couldn't finish my food, and soon, I couldn't even sit in the booth during the contractions. We called the doula, and she met me at the restaurant and drove me home. My husband and son stopped at the store before coming home, to get snacks and drinks for me. At one point, while I was on my hands and knees during a contraction, I said that I wished I'd vacuumed the carpet. As soon as that contraction was over, my doula got me into a bathtub of warm water—and vacuumed my house." —Melody, Washington

and labor and delivery care. Midwives are trained to care for normal, noncomplicated pregnancies. While midwives are fully capable of delivering a baby in an emergency situation, they are not trained to deal with high-risk pregnancies. A midwife watches her client for any warning signs, and if a patient becomes high risk, the midwife will refer her patient to an obstetrician.

As we have mentioned several times, doulas do not provide any prenatal care or labor and delivery medical care. Perhaps doulas and midwives are mistaken as being one and the same because they both approach pregnancy and birth as a normal event, as opposed to a medical event.

Of course, a midwife's philosophies will be affected by the hospital or birth center she works in and her training background. Whether you decide to hire a midwife or obstetrician, interview them and make sure you're compatible. You may be surprised to find an obstetrician who treats pregnancy and birth as normal events and takes a watchman's approach, or you may find a midwife who chooses to use many interventions. Neither a midwife nor an obstetrician can be viewed as the "best" choice.

Some midwives will meet with you during active labor and act as your birth coach. Even so, the midwife, especially during the birth, will need to provide medical care and supervision. She will not be there for you emotionally 100 percent of the time, and she cannot physically support you if you're in the process of pushing out the baby. If you hire a midwife who plans to support you during active labor, ask her what she thinks about doulas. Ask her exactly how much labor support she plans on providing and how long she plans on staying with you during labor and birth. She may even be able to give you names and numbers of local doulas.

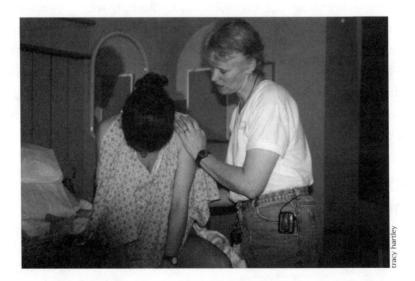

FIGURE 6.2. While a doctor will be in and out of the room, your doula will be by your side throughout labor. Doula tracy hartley of BestDoulas.com supports this second-time mother as she progresses quickly through labor.

If you have hired a midwife who does not stay with you during active labor, or who catches babies in a birth center or hospital, then your need for a doula is the same as a mother who hires an obstetrician. Just as obstetricians are only with you for a few moments during the entire labor, midwives who work with many women at once or who do not offer birth-coaching services to their clients are also busy and only present for a few moments.

"Some midwives work very similarly to doulas once the woman hits the labor and delivery door," explains Sarah Krauskopf, a registered nurse and montrice. "However, I have yet to see one [meet their patient at] home. That's something the mom needs to know. Also, most midwives do not labor-sit as long as a doula does. They are in and out but more present than a doctor."

As with an obstetrician, let your midwife know at a prenatal appointment that you plan to hire a doula. If she seems opposed to the idea, try to find out why she's hesitant. Ask your doula to come meet your midwife at a prenatal appointment, and talk over any concerns. As mentioned in the section on obstetricians, if your midwife is negative about your doula, you will need to make a choice. It's never too late to switch care providers. If your midwife's concerns are specific to the particular doula you hired, find out why she is concerned. If her concerns are valid, you may consider hiring a different doula. Ask your midwife if she has anyone to suggest.

# Homebirth, Hospitals, and Birthing Centers

Even before you decide which care provider to hire, you should decide where you'd like to give birth. You may find the perfect caregiver, but if she works in a hospital that has policies that are not in tune with your birth philosophies, your birth experience may be less than ideal.

## HOMEBIRTH

Homebirth may be the right choice for you if:

- You have a normal and healthy pregnancy.
- You are committed to giving birth without pain medication.
- You trust in the birth process.
- You wish to rest at home, in your own bed, after the birth.

If you'd like to give birth at home, then you'll want to

- Find out what the local laws are regarding homebirth.
- Find a midwife or physician that offers homebirth services.
- Prepare for normal childbirth by reading, practicing relaxation techniques, and attending a childbirth education class. Be sure to educate yourself in the procedures and interventions of any hospital that you may be transferred to, in the case of an emergency.
- Read as much as you can about preparing for a homebirth. Check out www.motheringmagazine.com for more information and support forums on homebirth.
- Hire a doula for the birth, a postpartum doula for your first days and weeks, and enlist the help of friends or a babysitter for your older children.

## HOSPITAL BIRTH

Hospital birth may be the right choice for you if:

- You have a high-risk pregnancy or any medical problems that makes birthing in a hospital necessary.

- You are not sure if you want a pain-medication–free birth.
- You feel safer in the hospital environment.
- You wish to rest in a hospital environment for a day or two after the birth.

To find a hospital that is best for you, you'll want to

- Call the nurse manager of the hospital and ask her what their policies are regarding fetal monitoring, walking around during birth, having a doula present for the birth, eating and drinking, laboring or birthing in water, IV usage, photography, or any other important questions you have.
- Call the nurse manager of the postpartum unit and ask about their rooming-in policies, if they require taking the baby to the nursery at any time during your stay, if breastfeeding support or bottlefeeding support is available, and any other important questions.
- Find out what percentage of the patients use epidural anesthesia or require cesarean section.
- Schedule a tour of the hospital's labor and delivery unit and postpartum unit. Talk to the staff; ask any questions you have.
- Find a midwife or obstetrician who delivers babies in that hospital.
- Prepare for childbirth by educating yourself. Be sure to educate yourself in the various interventions and medications that may be offered in a hospital setting.
- Hire a doula for the birth and a postpartum doula for your first days and weeks home. Arrange for a babysitter to watch your older children while you're in the hospital.

## BIRTH CENTER

A birth center may be the right choice for you if:

"I was very pleased with my first birth experience with a midwife. She never left my side and helped with labor by making suggestions to change positions, use the shower, etc. She encouraged me through praise and reassurance during the hardest part of my labor. She also kept the room quiet and calm and kept away unnecessary medical interventions. I assumed my second experience would be very similar since I was once again using a midwife. We had moved to a new state at the time of my second pregnancy, so I was not able to use my first midwife. I discovered through the labor and delivery of my second child that not all midwives are like my first. My second labor and delivery ended up with an epidural and me laboring on my back. My midwife was rarely even in the room until it was time to push.

"After finding myself pregnant for the third time, I decided to do some research. I had heard of doulas before but didn't see the need for one due to my belief that all midwives would play the same role as my first. I discovered through my research both over the Internet and with phone calls that midwives (at least near where I live) are just another person on the medical staff. Through further research I came to realize that my first midwife had played the role of both doula and midwife. So I decided I needed to look into hiring a doula." —Tiffany, Georgia

- You have a normal, healthy pregnancy.
- You are committed to giving birth without pain medication.
- You want a family-centered birth with more freedom, little or no intervention, and access to birthing pools.

- You feel safer in a birth center than at home.
- You wish to be at home with your newborn within six to twelve hours after the birth.

To find a birth center, you'll want to

- Ask local doulas or midwives for the nearest birth center locations. You can also contact the National Association for Childbearing Centers at 215-234-8068, or visit their homepage at www.birthcenters.org.
- Call the birth center and ask if the birth attendants are licensed healthcare providers, if the center is accredited by the Commission for the Accreditation of Birth Centers, how complications are dealt with, and when and how transfers to hospitals are made. For a list of more detailed questions to ask, visit www.birthcenters.org.
- Tour the birth center; ask the staff questions.
- Find a midwife or obstetrician who delivers babies in that hospital.
- Prepare for normal childbirth by reading, practicing relaxation techniques, and attending a childbirth education class. Be sure to educate yourself in the procedures and interventions of any hospital that you may be transferred to, in the case of an emergency.
- Hire a birth doula for labor and a postpartum doula for your first days and weeks home. Insurance may cover postpartum care if you are dismissed early from the birth center, so ask the birth center about this option.

CHAPTER 7

# Hiring a Labor Doula

WHEN I BEGAN SEARCHING for a doula, there were a few things I knew I wanted. I wanted a doula who had given birth normally, ideally to more than one or two kids. I wanted a doula with experience in hospital births and someone who received training from one of the doula organizations. I needed a doula who was comfortable with my spiritual but practical approach to birth, and someone who understood that my husband would not take an active role in supporting me physically during labor.

As far as services were concerned, I wanted a doula who would attend me at home, as I planned on laboring as long as possible outside of the hospital environment. I didn't care about the extras, like photography or a birth story, or alternative approaches to pain management, like aromatherapy. Obviously, I needed a doula who was available for my due date. Last, but not least, I needed someone who could arrange a payment plan and whose fee was within my financial reach.

I contacted at least fifteen different doulas via email or telephone. Once I found a few doulas who fit my requirements, I arranged interviews, looking to see if my husband and I felt comfortable with the doula, if our personalities clicked, and if I could see myself laboring with her as my support. I interviewed two women and hired the second doula I met.

Your experience may vary. What I looked for in a doula may or may not be important to you. If you're giving birth at home or in a birth center, experience with hospitals may be irrelevant. You may not need to speak with as many doulas as I did; perhaps the first doula you meet will be a perfect match. Your childbirth educator may offer to attend you, or you may have a friend who's a doula. (However, don't feel obligated to hire her just because she is your friend!)

Whatever your experience, there are a few important steps to finding and hiring the right doula for you.

## What Do You Want?

Before you begin searching for a doula, it's important to think over your reasons for hiring one. Personally, I wanted someone who had been in my shoes before and survived. Essentially, I wanted someone to stand nearby and "guard" my birth—which is exactly what my doula did.

I didn't need a lot of active support from my doula. She spent most of my labor giving me short bits of advice over the phone, before I asked her to come to my house, and when I did ask her to come, she held my hand and wiped my brow with a cool cloth. She also made sure I was always comfortable, looking for extra pillows and helping me clean up after vomiting. It may seem like my doula didn't do much, but I know I could not have labored so calmly without her. Her mere presence lent me the strength I needed to labor on my own, without medication, and that was what I wanted from a doula.

While you don't need to have a definite idea of what you want from your birth, you do need to consider what's most important to you. Here are a few questions to ponder before you start calling people:

### A BIRTHING MOMENT . . .

"My doula helped so much. I had a 34-hour labor and she was there for about 30 of those. She did massage, aromatherapy for my nausea, hot and cold compresses on my back. I had an agonizing back labor and was in excruciating pain for a lot of my labor. She helped me move labor along by helping me get in different positions to bring on contractions. She cleaned up my vomit and wiped the blood from between my legs. She walked the halls and stairwell of the hospital with me. She spent a good deal of my labor applying counterpressure to my back and teaching my husband to do the same. I noticed that my husband started emulating the things she was doing, and we all worked as a team. She also provided me with incredible emotional support. She held my hand and kept eye contact with me. When I was starting to lose it, she brought me back. She distracted me from how long everything was taking. I remember at one point saying, 'I can't do this.' She responded, 'You're doing it.' I thought, 'My God, she's right, I am!' That really helped me."
—Ann Marie, Indiana

- Why do you want a doula?
- What type of childbirth education have you received and how do you view the process of labor and birth?
- Do you want a doula to provide a refresher or private childbirth education classes? (You may need to pay an extra fee.)
- Are there any religious considerations that may arise during birth?
- Do you want a doula who will take photographs or video? Help with birth art or write a birth story?

- Do you prefer a doula who is trained or experienced with alternative pain management techniques, like acupressure, aromatherapy, herbal remedies, water birth, or others?
- Are you planning on getting an epidural? Do you want a doula who has supported women who have chosen this option before?
- Do you want a doula who is willing to provide labor support at home?
- Do you want a doula who will help you find a care provider or help you arrange a homebirth by putting you in contact with local midwives?
- How much are you able to pay, and do you have an upper limit? (The average total fee for an experienced doula is $400, but fees range from $250 up to $1,000, depending on area of the country and experience.)

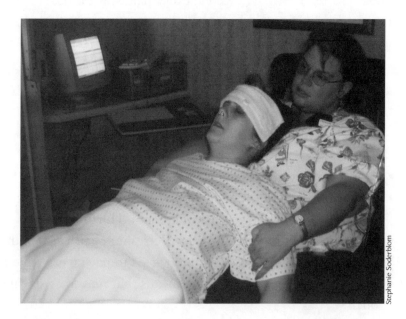

FIGURE 7.1. A doula provides continuous support to her client.

- How far away are you willing to seek out a doula? Do you have fast labors, and therefore, prefer that the doula lives within 30 minutes? Or are you willing to look within an hour's driving distance?

Decide what is most important to you, and what you consider optional desires. I knew I could not pay more than $600 for a doula, so anyone who charged more than $600 was automatically not an option. (Of course, I always asked if they had a sliding scale or were willing to barter to make up the part of the fee I could not pay—more about this later.) While I wanted a doula who had given birth before and was certified with a national doula organization, I was flexible on these terms. I would not consider, however, a doula who was not willing to support me at home. (Some doulas will only meet with the woman after she's been admitted to the hospital or birth center.)

After speaking with a few doulas, you may change your mind about what you originally intended for your birth experience. That's fine. Since education is a part of your doula's service, it's logical to assume that you may reconsider your approach to birth. Your main goal in finding a doula is trying to match your personality and general outlook. All the details will fall into place if you can find someone you feel comfortable with.

# Where to Look

Now that you have a general idea of what you're looking for, the next step is to call some doulas and arrange interviews. Where should you look to find a doula?

Friends, family, or your childbirth educator are good places to start. Ask if they know of any doulas; and if they personally used her services, ask what they thought. Keep in mind, however, that what they tell you is just their personal opinion. The doula who

"I think my doula chose me. I was about six months pregnant, and though I was talking a lot about my intention to hire a doula, I had yet to do anything about it. Then a friend gave my name to an old friend of hers who is a doula. My friend is legally blind, yet Artie, my friend's doula, had coached her in African dancing, among other things. She said, 'I would trust Artie to lead me through anything.' So she passed on my number, and Artie called me. We talked for a while on the phone, and I got a very positive feeling from her. Her first baby had been caesarean, yet the next four were vaginal deliveries! By the end of the conversation, she said, 'I would like to be your doula. When can we meet?' After I hung up the phone, I told my husband, 'I think our doula just chose us!'" —Megan, Minnesota

they describe as wonderful may not be the right doula for you; or vice versa, the doula who they thought was so-so may be the best one for you.

No matter what report they give, good or bad, get the number and give a call. Unless they tell you something serious, like she didn't show up for the birth or return calls, it's worth calling and speaking with her. The worst that will happen is you will decide not to meet her in person.

### DOULA ORGANIZATIONS

Almost all doula-certifying organizations provide referral services. Many have this information available on their websites, and sometimes a link to the doula's website or an email address is provided. Here are the top doula organizations, in alphabetical order:

ALACE—The Association of Labor Assistants and Childbirth
    Educators
P.O. Box 382724
Cambridge, MA 02238
617-441-2500
email: alacehq@aol.com
www.alace.org

BBI—Birth and Bonding International
1126 Solano Ave.
Albany, CA 94706
510-527-2121
email: bbint@flash.net
www.birthbonding.org

Birthing from Within
123 Wellesley SE
Albuquerque, NM 87106
505-254-4884
email: contact@birthingfromwithin.com
www.birthpower.com

Birth Works
P.O. Box 2045
Medford, NJ 08055
888-TO-BIRTH (862-4784)
email: info@birthworks.org
www.birthworks.org

CAPPA—Childbirth and Postpartum Professional Association
P.O. Box 491448
Lawrenceville, GA 30043
888-548-3672
email: info@cappa.net
www.cappa.net

CEF—Childbirth Enhancement Foundation
1004 George Ave.
Rockledge, FL 32955
321-631-9977
email: info@cefcares.org
www.cefcares.org

DONA—Doulas of North America
P.O. Box 626
Jasper, IN 47547
801-756-7331
email: doula@dona.org
www.dona.org

ICEA—The International Childbirth Education Association
P.O. Box 20048
Minneapolis, MN 55240
952-854-8660; 800-827-ICEA
email: info@icea.org
www.icea.org

You may want to call your local maternity hospitals or birth centers and ask if they have a referral list for doulas, or your midwife or obstetrician may be helpful in finding a doula. Also, La Leche League leaders are often familiar with the local birth community. To find a La Leche League leader, call 800-LALECHE or visit their website at www.lalecheleague.org.

## DOULA WEB SITES
There are several Web sites that maintain searchable doula databases. Many of these sites provide doulas the opportunity to list their Web sites and email addresses and describe their services, training, or experience. Here are a few of the larger sites:

A BIRTHING MOMENT . . .

"My doula kept talking to me in a low calm tone and telling me to visualize the pain going down my leg and into the floor and white light and energy coming up through the other leg and washing the pain out and down through the first leg. The soothing words and the sound of her voice helped a lot. There were times my husband said that if someone had walked in they would have thought I was sleeping, that I was so calm looking. She also really encouraged me to moan and groan and let it be deep and pushing. It worked great since I wouldn't have been comfortable screaming and yelling and it was a good way to release the tension." —Harmony, Ohio

About.com's Pregnancy Resources
www.pregnancy.about.com/health/pregnancy/library/local/
bllocalindex.htm

Birth Partners—Doulas
www.birthpartners.com

Doula Network
www.doulanetwork.com

DoulaWorld.com
www.doulaworld.com

Life Directory
www.lifedirectory.com

The Labor of Love Pregnancy and Parenting Search Engine
www.thelaboroflove.com/websearch/links/Services/Doulas

In some parts of the country, finding a doula may be difficult. In this case, consider calling childbirth educators. Many instructors offer doula services to their students, but they may not advertise themselves as doulas. It's worth calling to ask if they'd provide doula services to a non-student. See appendix E for childbirth education contact information.

# Avoiding the "Wrong" Doula

Unfortunately, not every woman who calls herself a doula should be one. As in every profession, there are doulas out there who either work for the wrong reasons, have personal agendas, or are irresponsible. Marilee of Illinois had a negative experience with her doula. She met hers at a doula tea, a gathering that brings several doulas and mothers together to meet and ask questions, that was sponsored by her childbirth educator.

"We asked lots of questions about their techniques. We had to take cost into consideration since my husband and I didn't have much money," Marilee explains. "We chose our doula based on her answers to our questions, and the fee she was charging. She was a doula-in-training, so her fee was lower than an experienced doula."

Marilee decided to hire the doula on the spot. She met the doula one more time to discuss birth plans. Unfortunately, Marilee's health took a turn for the worse and she was restricted to bed rest. "So, there I was, at home and in bed, lying on my side for most of the day," she explains, "only getting up to use the bathroom. I called my doula, who returned my call once. She never followed up to check on me, she never came over to see how I was doing . . . nothing."

"Four weeks prior to my due date, I went back to my OB for a checkup," Marilee continues. "My blood pressure skyrocketed, and I was told that I had eclampsia. They admitted me immediately and gave me drugs to induce labor." Marilee called her doula and her best friend, Jenny, and met them at the hospital.

"I was having contractions, and the doula was helping me try and manage the pain with some imaging and focusing techniques," she says. "Things seemed to kind of spiral out of control, however. Then, they started talking about an emergency c-section because things weren't progressing quickly enough. I opted then for an epidural, which helped me to sleep a little.

"While all this was going on, Jenny, my husband, and the doula were talking. The doula was telling us about her marriage and how she and her husband didn't have any children yet because her husband was impotent! She went on and on about his issues with sex, and the fact that in all their years of marriage they only had intercourse twice! I really couldn't believe I was hearing this!

"About three hours after receiving the epidural," Marilee continues, "the doctor checked to see how I was progressing. I wasn't, so they gave me one more dose of the medicine and said that if I didn't start to progress within a half hour, they would have to do the c-section. I told my husband to go with Jenny to grab something to eat at the Burger King across the street from the hospital. The doula took this opportunity to leave. . . . She said she had to make her husband dinner. While they were gone, I dilated. Luckily, Jenny and my husband were only across the street. They came back just in time to help me through about an hour of contractions . . . then pop! Hannah popped out into her daddy's arms. The doula, however, didn't get back until way after Hannah was born."

Marilee's doula did visit her once in the hospital after the birth, but the doula never contacted her again. Obviously, Marilee's doula experience was anything but positive. I asked Marilee what she would advise mothers to do, to avoid a negative experience. The following tips are based on her advice:

- *Call references!* "I failed to interview any of the women whose births our doula attended and that was my biggest mistake," says Marilee. "When I was searching for a daycare provider for my daughter, you can be certain that I thoroughly checked out references. Checking references is vital prior to hiring anyone." If a doula will not provide previous references, or claims that no one will allow her to give their names and phone numbers, consider that a red flag.

- *If your doula is certified, check with the certification agency.* Just email the organization that the doula claims to be certified by and ask if she is certified and if there have been any negative reports on her.

---

### 🐦 A BIRTHING MOMENT . . .

"I was a gestational surrogate for dear friends—their child was conceived through IVF. I was delivering the genetic child of my friends, who were both in attendance. The mother-to-be sometimes gets woozy, so we had decided early on that when the time came for the baby to be born, she would sit to the side in the rocking chair. . . . I had the intended father holding one of my legs, and my doula helping with the other. The intended mom was [sitting in the rocking chair], and then suddenly, she was standing next to me! I was so worried about her, but her son was crowning and she couldn't wait to see him! The baby seemed to be born quickly and watching her watch me give birth to her son was beyond words. The joy I saw on her face, and the tears streaming, was amazing! As her son was placed on my stomach, she just cried and put her hands on her cheeks . . . leading my doula to take her hand and gently put it on the baby's back, saying "Touch your baby!" Those few moments are etched in my mind, showing how a doula helps all women becoming mothers —beautiful!" —Staci, Colorado

- *Trust your instincts.* Even if you already hired the doula and signed a contract, back out if you think something is not right. You may lose your down payment, but a negative birth experience (or worse) is not worth saving the money.
- *If you are planning to hire a doula who is pursuing certification, ask for her doula trainer's or mentor's phone number.* Ask if the trainer or mentor thinks your doula is professional and if she has any reservations. If the doula-in-training has not attended any trainings or births, then check with previous employers.
- *Take the time to interview each doula carefully before deciding who to hire, and speak with them more than once.* I know during pregnancy you're tired and not in the mood to call or meet with many people, but this is the birth of your child and the birth of you becoming a mother. Don't feel pressured by anyone, take your time, and start looking for a doula early in pregnancy so you'll feel at ease with the process of hiring one.

# Interviewing

Before you actually call someone, you'll want to write down what questions you'd like to ask. (See appendix 1 for an interview guide.) Personally, I write down exactly what I want to say, so I don't jumble my words or forget to mention something important. Good questions to ask include:

- Are you available for my due date?
- What kind of training and experience have you had?
- What is your personal childbirth philosophy?
- What services do you provide?
- Are you willing to meet with me at home before I go to the hospital/birth center?

"In Bloomington we have an amazing community resource called Bloomington Area Birth Services (BABS). It was founded by a very devoted and inspiring woman named Georg'ann Cattelona. I visited on a Wednesday morning, which is a gathering time for new parents, their babies, and pregnant women. I was stunned that morning to discover almost ten mothers with their babies, all crowded into a relatively small room chatting, sharing stories, and caring for their little ones. In the middle of all the activity sat Georg'ann. I asked her about the doula services offered by BABS, and she gave me all the information and mentioned that there were a number of women working as doulas in town. She encouraged me to interview some of them to find the right match for me and my husband. By the end of our conversation, I was pretty confident that the right match was Georg'ann, so I asked her if she would be available for an interview. We set it up and a few days later, my husband and I met with her. We both agreed that we felt very comfortable with her and didn't feel the need to look any further." —Andrea, Indiana

- What do you charge for your services? Do you offer payment plans?
- Do you have any clients I can call as references?
- Can we meet for a face-to-face interview? Do you charge a fee for this meeting?

The doula will let you know if she is available and answer your queries, or she may tell you she's booked for that month and offer names of other local doulas. She may ask you to call her back another time or ask for your number. Be prepared to write down any information.

If you like the answers she gives, you may decide to meet in person. Don't feel pressured to schedule an interview after one phone conversation. You may want to call a few doulas, get an idea for what's out there, and then, call back your favorites. Or you may love the first person you speak to!

While some doulas will meet you at your home for the interview, I suggest meeting in a public place. I'll admit I met with one doula in my house, but I'm not sure how wise a decision that was. Better to play it safe. You can meet in a coffee shop, library, bookstore, or park. The doula may know a good place to meet, so you may ask her for suggestions. Try to arrange a time when your husband can come along. Even if he can't stay for the entire interview, he should at least meet her and say hello.

Bring your list of questions or concerns you formulated when considering what you're looking for in a doula. Here are some questions to consider:

- Why did you become a doula?
- What is your personal experience with childbirth?
- Tell me what your most challenging labor support experience was.
- What do you think about the use of medication during labor?
- What is your experience with hospital births/homebirths/birth center births?
- What happens if you cannot attend the birth?
- Will you take pictures of the birth or video? Do you charge extra for this service?
- Do you have backup? Under what circumstances do you call her? Can we meet with her?
- How do you arrange payment for services? How much do we need to pay up front?
- Do you accept credit cards? Personal checks?
- Do you have a contract?

These are just examples of the questions you may want to ask. Keep in mind that the most experienced doula, or the doula with the most impressive service package, is not necessarily the best doula for your birth. Ask yourself: Am I comfortable with this person? Does she seem like someone I can get along with? Do I agree with her philosophy? Does she seem pushy or judgmental? Does she listen while I speak, or does she look like she's just thinking of what to say next? Is she confident? Knowledgeable?

Go with your gut feeling. Maybe she offers all the services you want and seems like a nice person, but you just don't like her. It happens. Her voice annoys you or your husband does not feel right about her. Then she's not the doula for you. It's not politically correct, but remember you're trying to find someone to attend one of the most important moments of your life. You want someone who you like, not someone who makes you feel uncomfortable.

After your interview, you may decide to sign a contract right away, or you may want to meet a few more people. Personally, I waited until after the interview to talk it over with my husband privately. I called my doula back the same day as the interview so that she could reserve the two weeks surrounding my due date.

> "Doulas are as different as people within any profession. Some have more education and enthusiasm than others. Some are certified, some aren't. Some doulas are laid-back and some are more high-energy. We tried to find a person like ourselves."
> —Kris, Washington

## Contracts and Payment

At the interview, you'll talk about payment for services. Ask your doula to provide in writing her services and payment terms. While not all doulas require their clients to sign a contract, I believe it is best for both parties. A contract protects the doula and you by explaining in writing exactly what the doula's services include and what her services do not include, by detailing the payment terms, and by outlining the client's and doula's responsibilities.

## CONTRACTS

When reading over your doula's contract, or writing one together, the following questions should be addressed:

- What services will the doula provide?
- What services are not provided by the doula? (For example: A doula does not provide prenatal care or midwifery services.)
- How many prenatal and postnatal meetings are included in the labor doula's service package? If I'd like to meet additional times, will there be an additional cost? How much?
- What are the fees for each service? (For example: labor doula service $400, videography $30, and so on.)
- At which point during labor will the doula attend us, and how does the doula want us to contact her? (For example: phone, pager, and so on.)
- What if I call and I am not in labor? (Some doulas charge a small fee, referred to as a "false alarm" fee. Others consider false alarms to be a part of the regular doula service.)
- What amount am I required to pay in order for the doula to hold my due date on her calendar?
- If a payment schedule has been negotiated, when are the payments due? What happens if the payments are late?
- If I decide to break the contract, how much will the doula refund, or how much do I owe the doula for holding my space and spending time meeting with me?

- If the doula decides to break the contract, how much will the doula refund of my payment? Is she required to find another doula who will provide services?
- Under what circumstances will my doula call her backup? How will the payment schedule play out if the doula does call her backup?

Be sure to read through the contract, and don't be afraid to ask questions. If you disagree with anything, mention your concerns. Unless you have hired a labor doula service that is run by a larger agency, the contract is usually negotiable. One contract I reviewed stated that the client owes the doula the full fee in the event that the doula does not make it to the birth, for example, in the case of an unusually fast birth. I negotiated that a lower fee should be charged, perhaps half of the regular fee, and the doula readily agreed and had no problem changing the contract.

## PAYMENT

Doula fees vary according to region, services provided, and the experience and training of the doula. Flat fees range anywhere from $100 up to $1,500, and the average fee is $375 for a certified and moderately experienced doula. Some charge an hourly rate. Usually, doulas-in-training charge less than $200 and doulas who have received certification charge no less than $300. I discovered in my search for a doula that the average doula fee in New England is closer to $450, and I know that some doulas in San Francisco charge $1,000 for basic doula service. When you speak to doulas on the phone or via email, ask about their rates to get a better idea of your area's average.

Most doulas require a down payment along with the signed contract before they will hold your due date. This fee may be half of the doula's full price or a mere fraction. Other doulas ask to be paid in full right from the start.

The majority of doulas are interested in making their service affordable for you. If you find a doula you'd like to have at your birth, but her price is out of your range, tell her. Try to find a payment plan that will help you afford her services, or ask if she's willing to negotiate her fee. I paid $450 for my doula and spread out the payments over several months, paying 1/3 of the payment every four weeks. The doula should receive her full payment no later than your due date. After the baby is born, you'll be busy mothering your new child and paying your doula will be far from your mind.

Some doulas offer a sliding-scale fee. They may tell you that they charge anywhere from $350 up to $450, with most clients paying the average of those two numbers. In this case, you may be able to choose where in that range you'd like to pay. Other doulas charge according to the client's income.

Possibly, the doula who you just love may not be within your financial means. She may not be able to adjust her fees to your needs, but she can refer you to other doulas with similar philosophies. Don't be embarrassed to ask for referrals; doulas are used to giving out referrals and will not be offended.

> "Our doula told us that she was still trying to get her three births for her certification; she still needed two. [We negotiated her fee to] a third of what the going rate was, and I made her some hand-painted Ukrainian style eggs, which she fell in love with, as payment."
> —Harmony, Ohio

## ALTERNATIVE PAYMENT METHODS

Cash is not the only option for payment. Bartering for doula services is also viable, for those willing to work together in finding an appropriate deal. Usually bartering is used when a family cannot afford to pay the full fee. Haircuts, babysitting, homemade quilts, educational classes, fresh veggies and herbs from gardens—all of these have been used as barter for doula services. Some barter the entire fee or use bartering as a supplement to cash. Whether you pay in cash or through an alternative means, make sure everything is in writing.

Whatever you intend to barter, it should be equal to the cost of the services. For example, let's say she charges the average $375. If you'd be willing to barter babysitting services plus pay $100, then you'd need to babysit her kids for $275 worth. If a private sitter is paid around $10 per hour, then that would be about 27 hours of babysitting.

Of course, your doula will let you know what she considers a fair item or service to barter. It's best to provide the bartered service or item before you give birth because, as I mentioned earlier, after the baby comes, you'll be very busy.

Another alternative: Consider including doula services on your holiday or baby shower wish list. Perhaps a few friends or relatives could contribute to a doula fund.

## Third-Party Reimbursement

You may not have to pay out-of-pocket for your doula. Insurance companies are beginning to cover their services. Doulas save insurance companies thousands of dollars by lowering c-section rates, epidural and drug usage; helping moms breastfeed (which lowers doctor visits); empowering women to have positive birth experience (which lessens postpartum depression); and more. Unfortunately, some companies do not realize how much a doula is worth, or do not realize there is a demand for doula care coverage.

First, have your doula create an invoice that lists her name and company, her credentials and certification number, her address, phone number, tax or social security number, and the amount being billed. The invoice should also include your information: your name and address, birthday, social security number, date and location of services provided, due date, and insurance policy number. If the insurance is provided by someone other than yourself, for example, through your husband's work, then mention his contact information as well.

The invoice should also contain the proper diagnostic codes and services-rendered codes. The codes were originally developed by the Health Care Financing Administration, and while they may change from year to year, they are usually the same. For the diagnosis, the invoice should list diagnostic code V22.2, which is for intrauterine pregnancy. For the services rendered, you'd most likely want to use CPT code 99499 Evaluation and Management Services. If you're not sure what code to use, call the insurance company and ask. Be sure to note on the invoice that the services rendered were prenatal consultation and labor support.

If you are denied your claim, reapply and include a letter from your doula outlining the benefits of doula care. Most insurance companies will assign a case worker to your claim if you appeal, and this gives you a chance to explain why they should cover doula care. Also, write a letter explaining how the doula helped you, and most importantly, how the use of a doula saved the insurance company money. Did you give birth without medication? Did you avoid a c-section? All of this should be mentioned in the letter. Try to call wherever you gave birth and ask them how much they charge for an epidural, narcotics, or a c-section birth. Include those prices, if they apply, in your letter. For a sample invoice and sample reimbursement letter, please see appendix 2 of this book.

Even if you believe that your insurance company will turn your claim down, apply anyway. If more people apply for insurance coverage for doulas, then the companies will be more inclined to cover such care. Insurance companies, like all businesses, are influenced by consumer demand.

Flexible spending accounts may also be used for doula care. Check with your employer or your partner's employer for more information.

# Free Doula Programs

If hiring a private doula is beyond your financial reach, look into local doula volunteer programs. Hospitals throughout the country are setting up doula programs, offering patients labor support services for free or at a reduced rate, $50 or less. Call local hospitals and speak to either the labor and delivery department or the education department.

While doula volunteer programs are great if you cannot afford to hire a private doula, there are disadvantages. One issue is that the volunteer is working for the hospital, so she may not be free to say or

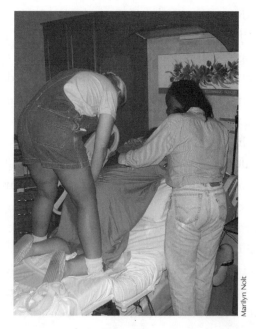

FIGURE 7.2. A doula applies pressure to the back of a laboring mom. This is a great technique for back labor.

encourage certain things for political reasons. Another consideration is that many programs do not allow you to choose who will attend the birth. The doula who happens to be on-call when you go into labor may or may not be someone you'd choose if you had chosen to hire privately.

The most significant problem with some hospital doula programs is that the doulas may not be able to provide continuous support, from the time you are admitted until just after the birth. The doula may need to leave when their on-call hours are up, so you may lose your support while in transition. It's difficult to redevelop trust with another doula at an intense time like this, and the research on doulas shows that intermittent support does not produce as impressive results when compared to continuous support.

Many hospital programs remedied these concerns and offer excellent doula services. When you call the hospital for information on their doula program, you'll want to ask:

- What kind of training do the doulas receive?
- What do I need to do in order to sign up for the doula program?
- Will I be given any help in writing a birth plan? Do I need to submit a birth plan to the doula program?
- Will I be able to meet with the doula who will attend me during birth before I go into labor? May I meet any of the doulas who volunteer in your program beforehand?
- At which point will the doula attend me? Can I ask for doula support before being admitted to the hospital? How long after the birth will the doula stay with me?
- Will the same doula support me throughout the birth, even if my birth goes beyond her on-duty time?
- Are there any fees? When do I need to pay? Will my insurance cover the doula fees?

Danbury Hospital's doula program in Connecticut serves as the model for many volunteer programs throughout the United States. Their website contains a wealth of information and explains their program and its goals. You can visit the site at www.geocities.com/Wellesley/Garden/4022/dhdbegan.html.

Hospitals are not the only place to find free doula care. Another option is to hire a doula-in-training. Doulas who are seeking births to fulfill certification requirements may attend births for free or for a reduced fee. While they may not have varied experience, doulas-in-training who are seeking certification births have already attended trainings and read several books that are required for certification. Some have attended births as an observer or with a mentor.

Call local doulas to ask if they know of anyone looking for certification births. You can also call doula trainers from various organizations. If you visit the websites of the doula organizations and look for information on becoming a doula, you should be able to find contact information for doula trainers in your area. Call them and ask if they can recommend any of their students.

Be sure to check references. Even though a doula-in-training may not be able to provide names of former clients, she can provide names and numbers of people she came in contact with while training. For example, she may be able to give you the name and number of her doula trainer or of a childbirth education teacher she worked with. Don't hesitate to call former employers if she doesn't have any birth-related references to contact.

If you cannot find any hospital volunteer programs or find any doulas in training, try calling the Childbirth Enhancement Foundation at 321-631-9977. CEF specializes in community- and hospital-based doula programs and may be aware of smaller doula volunteer programs in your area.

## CHAPTER 8

# Two Beautiful Birth Stories

So NOW YOU KNOW what doulas do and how to hire one. The best way to understand how doulas help mothers during childbirth, besides experiencing it personally, is by reading birth stories.

Here are two beautiful ones. The first is by Georganne Hampton, with comments from her doula (*in italics*), about the homebirth of her daughter, Olivia Marie. In the second story, Sharon Quarrington, her husband Bruce Craig (in this font), and their doula (*in italics*) tell the birth story of their daughter, Kiera Elizabeth.

## OLIVIA MARIE'S BIRTH STORY

*As told by Georganne Hampton and her doula Danielle (in italic)*

I had never really given much thought to actually having a homebirth myself, but for some reason the thought kept tickling the back of my mind. My good friend and original doula mentor had a homebirth, and it was a great experience. I started to do a bit of research on the subject. The more I read, the more I thought of it as an actual possibility for me.

*Georganne had recently come to Oklahoma before she and [her husband] Justin decided to try to have their second child. I met her at our local doula group meeting. The next month, we were hosting an informational booth at a local Toys "R" Us, when we felt that we "clicked." Later that evening at the meeting she mentioned her need for a doula. I told her I would be honored to serve her at her birth. She told me of her plans to have a homebirth. No problem, she would be my second homebirth and my fourteenth client. As the months passed, I told her of my desire to meet with her and Justin. I felt that it was just as important for Justin to feel comfortable with me as she did, since this event would really be about the two of them, and the birth of their child. We met for an informal lunch date, and I passed Justin's approval.*

*Also, I was [pregnant] after a nine-year break, and I wanted to have a serious talk with Georganne. Because I would be so far along, I was afraid that I would not be physically able to serve her during labor. I wanted her to know that I would not be upset if she decided to ask another doula to attend her birth, but she had become emotionally attached to me by that time. I was not going to "abandon her." I asked her if there was anyone else that she felt comfortable with and suggested a backup person. She just happened to choose a doula (Eileen) that lived only five minutes away from me. So that was the plan.*

Monday, September 24, I was feeling miserable. I spent the day doing some laundry, a bit of housework, running around town paying bills, and sitting at my computer. I had all my birth supplies ready, my bedroom was newly cleaned, and the batteries in the camcorder were charged. . . . I felt ready. I thought that it would be soon but also knew that that could be wishful thinking. I had been patient and had tried to enjoy this last part of my pregnancy.

Around 10:00 P.M. Monday night, [my husband] Justin went to bed. I stayed up reading email. By then I was too excited to sleep. I thought, "Something might be going on." I don't know why I thought this. I was not having contractions. I just knew.

I felt nothing happening so I decided to go to bed and tried to sleep.

I woke up at around 1:00 A.M. Got up, went to the bathroom, got back in bed, and snuggled up to my 3-year-old. I woke up again and looked at the clock. 1:10 A.M. I was so irritated. I just wanted to get some rest. Got up, went to the bathroom, got back in bed, snuggled up to my 3-year-old, reached over him and patted my husband on the shoulder, went back to sleep.

Woke up again! Looked at the clock. 1:20 A.M. A light bulb went on in my head. Okay, 10 minutes apart. The contractions were not painful, just enough to wake me up. . . .

By about 3:00 A.M., the contractions were getting more noticeable. I woke up my husband Justin just enough to tell him that "today we will be having a baby."

By 4:30 A.M., I no longer wanted to be alone. I didn't know whether I should call [my midwife and doula] yet or not. I called Gail, my midwife. I told her the contractions were 7 minutes apart, lasting a minute in length. She said she was on her way. I called my main doula, Danielle, who had a 1½ hour drive to get here.

At first I was still puttering around the house between contractions. I was amazed how great I felt in between them. Justin cleaned up the living room and did some puttering himself. He made me some toast, as I was still hungry. I remember I ate a couple of bites and left the rest on the table.

When [my doula] Danielle walked in the door I started to cry. I guess it was relief. I was just so happy to see her, and I knew that she would understand my tears. She was able to help me get my focus back pretty quickly.

Labor progressed. What a packed sentence that is. It has so much meaning. My doulas and Gail kept me moving. I hated each time they told me to go to the bathroom. Sitting on the toilet was agony. I would practically run in there after a contraction was over, rip up my nightgown, and try to pee before the next contraction hit. A doula would have to accompany me. As soon as I was done, I would have to stand up to lean over the back of the toilet to finish the contraction that it would bring on. They were so powerful. These were the only contractions that really scared me.

I labored in the kitchen, straddling a chair with the turtle pillow over the back of it. Danielle would sit on her birth ball behind me giving me counterpressure and rubbing my back and shoulders. Eileen would grab my hand and squeeze the pressure point there. That was my "ritual." I would find myself waving my hand for her to grab when a contraction started.

I walked up and down my hallway, stopping for contractions to lean over my washer and dryer. I lay on my side in my bed when I felt the need to rest. I asked for a honey stick to boost my energy. My doulas were great about keeping me hydrated and kept bringing my water from room to room. They were my constant companions. My husband Justin did not want such an active role and needed to feel that he could come and go as he felt the need to. I never felt his absence though, thanks to my doulas.

My sister Char was my videographer. She did a terrific job in capturing the essence of my labor. I told her to make the video as graphic as my labor was. I could edit it for public viewing later. Avone, my niece, showed up. I was so happy that she was there to experience this beautiful part of birth. She kept some of my girlfriends online updated on my progress. They were so excited to get a play-by-play, and I printed it all up for Olivia's baby book.

All throughout labor we just visited. We chatted as if we were girlfriends at a slumber party. Sometimes we laughed and giggled. Sometimes we were silly.

*I remember Justin coming into the room to check on Georganne and saying, "I never imagined laughing would be a part of labor, this is good!"*

It's a very strange sensation to be laughing during transition. I remember thinking that it was so nice to have these women around me, taking care of me, comforting me. It felt so right. I also remember how nice Gail's cool hands felt against my hot skin as she gave me some pats of love and strength.

After a few hours of this, Gail thought we might want to break my water. I had had a bulging bag but now there was not that much water in front of the baby's head. I had been doing all this work just to push her through the bulge of water.

*This was not "wasted time." It was used to empower her. She was able to work through some of the issues that came up emotionally from her first birth. We talked about them, and she was able to move through it at her own pace.*

I told her I was scared. I did agree to it shortly thereafter though. I just needed a few minutes to prepare my mind for this last little bit. I appreciated that no one tried to talk me into something I was not ready for. I was afraid, but I was also afraid of getting tired and I was ready to get it done.

Gail broke my water, and it was clear. Great! That was a relief to me. I finally felt a small need to push. It was never an overwhelming need, but it was definitely there.

I gave birth with my torso propped up on pillows on my bed. I was not flat on my back, but slightly on my side. I didn't think I would birth in this position, but it really was the most comfortable for me at the time. It was nice to know that I could have stood on my head if that is what I felt the need to do.

As the contractions became more intense so did the attention directed towards me. Everyone was there, helping me, praying for me, giving me encouragement and praising my strength, lending me their strength to lean on when mine failed. It seemed a very momentous time.

Danielle reminded me to work with my body and let it open up. Gail used the crockpot with ginger root in it to keep the compresses warm. These felt good on my perineum. Danielle reminded me that I wanted to see and touch my baby as she was crowning. I reached down and felt that my daughter had hair. My doula made sure someone brought my mirror so I could see.

With my support team reminding me to push through the pain, I pushed that first scary push. Her head was born. Gail checked for a cord around her neck. She was good. My contractions stopped. We waited. We waited some more. Gail looked at her watch. I took a deep breath. I started to wonder how long was too long between contractions once the head is born. I asked if we were waiting too long. Gail calmly said we need to get her out pretty soon. Her shoulders did not rotate as they are supposed to do and that may have had something to do with this situation.

I could see in the mirror that my baby's face was getting pretty dark. I decided to go ahead and push without the help of contractions. I knew she needed to be born. I could feel it. I think my fear of her shoulders being born was the culprit that stopped my contractions, but I was not going to let that stop me of course. After getting some reassurance from my team, I pushed. I pushed again. My body took the hint and kicked in a helping hand.

*Yes, when Olivia did not rotate her shoulders everything stopped. I was so impressed with the midwife, Gail. She let Georganne talk about her fear and gave her time to get past it and use her maternal instincts to know when to push without letting panic set in.*

Later on video, I could see (and hear) that I had added grunting to my ohs. I did not realize it at the time. I guess I really was in labor land. One shoulder came out to the sound of my one and only yell. I tore. The other shoulder followed soon after. Then, at long last, her body, followed by a huge, forceful swoosh of water. Relief, concern, adrenalin, satisfaction, empowerment, success! I did it!

Gail wiped her face off and gently suctioned her with the bulb. She lifted her up to me. My doulas threw a warm towel from the dryer over both of us. I raised my nightgown so we could be skin to skin. I peeked at her face under the towel. What a beautiful person we had made.

Danielle asked if I wanted to check to make sure she was a girl. She was. Olivia Marie. 9 pounds even, 19½ inches long. Born at 11:43 A.M.

I did tear to muscle since her shoulders did not rotate. It healed fine, though it did take a bit longer than I thought it would.

Well, where to go from here? How do I continue a story that is the beginning of life? I guess I cannot in the written form. I can only love and care for my daughter as her life develops. Because of this wondrous birth, I was taught to trust my body again. In my last birth, I was 11 days late due to emotional dystocia, and was extremely ill with preeclampsia. I was induced because my body "just wouldn't work right and go into labor on its own," and I always felt that I was not being told the complete story when asking questions of my caregivers. No one told me I actually could birth a baby without drugs, and I was threatened during the pushing stage with vacuum extraction, if I did not get this baby out "right now."

I thought I had come to terms with things that had happened in my previous birth, and in fact had worked out some of that in my subconscious. Little did I know how much more work I had yet to do. Fortunately I had chosen the perfect group of people to help me on my way. What an awesome journey.

# Kiera Elizabeth's Birth Story

*As told by Sharon Quarrington* (in this font), *her husband Bruce Craig* (in this font), *and their doula Heather* (*in italic*)

## MIDNIGHT

As soon as I get into bed I feel a cramp, very similar to a menstrual cramp, which didn't strike me as odd, except that a few minutes later I got another, and then another. After the first three, I timed them with my clock radio at about 5 minutes apart. I figured I should stay in bed. They probably didn't mean anything, but if this was "it," I would need my sleep.

3:00 A.M.

I wasn't sure if the cramps were getting stronger or not, but I couldn't seem to focus on TV or writing any more. . . . I decided to run a tub and see if that would help. Before I got in the tub, Bruce woke up and checked in with me.

"Are you just having trouble sleeping or . . ?" he says.

"I'm not sure," I replied. "But I am having fairly regular cramps."

"How regular?"

"Oh about every 3 minutes."

"What?!"

I felt excited, relieved, and scared all at once or, in a quick rotating sequence. Five minutes apart had been in the labor books as the beginning of the real thing. This could be the real thing! I was beginning to wake up quickly.

Sharon wasn't sure if this was real although she thought it might be. She was pouring a bath when I got up. The hot water may have relaxed her and helped the contractions. I debated going back to bed and sleeping a little more until her labor increased, but the adrenalin was starting to rush through me.

Needless to say, he didn't go back to bed, but decided to stay up and try timing the cramps while I was in the tub. By 3:30 A.M., the cramps were definitely getting stronger, and we both knew that this was it! Those cramps were really contractions.

At about 4:00 A.M., the contractions were at the same rate, but getting more visibly painful. Sharon could not talk and had to take deep breaths as each one gripped her abdomen. It seemed very real, and I was becoming concerned. We talked about calling Heather, our doula, and the doctor.

Sharon hesitated at first, wanting to be certain. I was beginning to feel panicky and unsure of what to do to help her during the contractions. Each one seemed more painful, and she had more difficulty maintaining her breathing and calmness.

4:30 A.M.

The cramps were getting tougher. I had to stop and concentrate on breathing with each one, and I was losing my sense of humor. The time to call had come. I called the doctor first. She was already at the hospital; she listened to a contraction and said it was okay to come in.

I talked to Heather, our doula, and we discussed whether to go to the hospital or not and decided to stay home for a little bit longer. She was great, coaching me through the breathing on the phone while she got herself ready to come over. Bruce wasn't so sure we should wait. Heather suggested having a shower to see if that would ease the cramps. It didn't. They kept coming stronger and closer together. Only 2 to 3 minutes apart and lasting for 45 to 60 seconds.

I was outside the glass shower door feeling more and more uncertain about what to do to help. I couldn't get into a rhythm with the breathing. I was either too fast or too slow for Sharon. My coaching didn't seem to help. All I could do was stay close and try to comfort her.

5:15 A.M.

Our doula Heather arrived.

*When I arrived around 5:15 A.M., I almost drove right past the house. I stopped the car because I noticed it was the only house in the street with all the lights on!*

*Bruce let me in and we found Sharon out of the shower wearing a comfortable big shirt. The first thing we did was exchange comments on our new haircuts—mine chopped, hers permed! What an intro.*

*I began breathing with Sharon and asking what had been working and what she didn't like. She seemed to like to pull down during the peak of a contraction (poor shower curtain) and invariably her arms went up and she rose on her toes at the peak. I asked what would help, and she responded, "A trip to Bermuda!"*

*Her contractions, we discovered, were already strung together in clumps that sometimes never went away. This continued to frustrate her throughout the labor and her main complaint was, "It's not like in the book: They're supposed to give me a break!!"*

*Bruce established a regular beat of counting up to 20 and back down. We soon learned that although this seemed to help Sharon, the contractions didn't build slowly and peak around 20 or 40 seconds— they peaked quickly and took longer to subside.*

I was starting to get a little panicky at this point. I had expected the pain to be strong, but I hadn't expected it to be so persistent. It felt like someone had driven a steel bar through both my hips and was vibrating it while standing on my lower uterus. The pain rarely went away, and as each contraction subsided, I could feel the next one coming on. I needed all the help and support Bruce could give me and, as always, he was right there for me.

It was as if the contractions were ocean waves, and as each swell began, the short breaths enabled Sharon to start moving with it, and as it built and crested, she breathed faster and harder to stay on top. I felt relieved and de-cided to learn from Heather, so I could help Sharon. I could not have figured this out from the books. I felt a tremendous relief and appreciation for Heather's expertise and ability to step in and take action.

6:30 A.M.

Heather suggested it was time to think about going to the hospital as the contractions were only 2 minutes apart and were lasting 40 sec-onds. I wanted to stay home as long as possible since I wasn't sure I would be comfortable at the hospital. . . . I've always hated them.

By this point, any touch on my belly would initiate a contraction. I tried to change out of my nightshirt into a jogging suit, but I couldn't take the pain. Finally I found old ratty pink maternity overalls and slipped them on over my shirt. So much for my stylish entry into the hospital.

Bruce packed the car—two suitcases, a CD player, Heather's big blue birthing ball, the drink cooler, the camera, and the camcorder.

The car ride was a nightmare—a Jeep with no shocks and roads covered in streetcar tracks. I couldn't sit down, so I went the whole way standing in the front, leaning over the passenger seat, looking at Heather in the back who was still gamely coaching me through my breathing. Poor Bruce had the task of driving as quickly and smoothly as he could.

7:00 A.M.

We arrived at the hospital. Now all my distances were measured in contractions. It took two contractions to get to the front door and three more to get to the elevator—where a well-meaning woman put her hand on my arm to comfort me, I think, but she set off another contraction. Bruce disengaged her arm for me. I really wasn't thinking too clearly at this point. Three more contractions and we were at the maternity triage. As luck would have it, the hospital was full. Even triage had no room. Heather suggested they just admit us, but they wanted us to wait. Bruce tried valiantly to keep me breathing while we were in the waiting room.

I was beginning to sense the depth of the pain and felt a deep fear of how intense it was. I was able to help her with her breathing with more coaching from Heather. I felt good at being able to do something directly. I got Sharon's attention by getting in direct eye contact and close to her. I did better with the breathing, but still felt awkward.

I was really tired and tried sitting in the rocking chair, but again, the touch of the chair set off another set of contractions. It seemed like the only thing I could do was stand, and the only place I could be touched was on my hands.

7:30 A.M.

Dr. Sheppard arrived, and I think they booted some poor woman out of triage to let us in, because my contractions were obviously coming quickly and painfully. The doctor did an assessment and gave us good news—I was 6 centimeters dilated and 90 percent effaced! Hurray! It couldn't be long now, could it?

Dr. Sheppard explained the pain options—basically a narcotic or an epidural. I said no to both, but the narcotic was tempting. I'd really wanted a drug-free birth, but this pain seemed to be more than I could handle. With Heather and Bruce's encouragement, I decided to wait a little longer before making a decision on the narcotic.

We met our wonderful nurse Doris and, unknown to me, Heather gave Dr. Sheppard and Doris copies of my birth plan. They read it on the slow trip to the labor and delivery room.

When we got to the room, I went immediately to the shower, feeling sticky with blood from the exam and hoping the shower would ease the pain a bit. The shower was almost hypnotizing; the pain was stronger, but more bearable. Time seemed to stand still except for the water level that slowly rose in the tub, and the people that kept checking in on me.

*Bruce and I took turns coaching Sharon's breathing and concentration during this time. We couldn't get the tub to unplug, and in our concern for a flood, decided to move to the room next door. I announced our intention to move, but Sharon quickly pointed out that she had 2 inches before overflowing and wanted to stay longer.*

*The contractions seemed more continuous in the shower, and Sharon sounded different. She moaned almost continually, and yet at the same time, there seemed to be a certain comfort that kept her there for quite some time.*

8:30 A.M.

After I got out of the shower we talked with Dr. Sheppard about pain relief again. Again I was tempted by the narcotic, but I was worried that it might have some negative impact on the baby, so I decided to hang in just a little longer.

I could see the fetal monitor in the corner of the room and was worried that they would put it on me. I knew that if they tried to put the monitor belt around my belly it would be very painful, but Doris, our nurse, was wonderful; she knew I wouldn't be able to sit still for it and simply placed the paddle that they used to hear the heartbeat on my belly whenever I was close enough. I guess they didn't need to check for contractions, they were pretty obvious.

All my carefully packed comfort items—the soft music, the aromatherapy ring, the frozen juices, and the books on labor positions—none of them mattered now. The only comfort items that mattered were people: Bruce, Heather, and Doris were all that could help now.

Once the doula and Doris had taken a good look at the cord blood kit we brought, Dr. Sheppard headed home for a shower. She'd already been at the hospital all night, and we were her fifth delivery. I was at a really low point. I'd been hoping the doctor would stay and the baby would arrive soon, but when she left saying it would be hours before the baby came, I was devastated. I wasn't sure I could stand this pain for many more minutes, much less for hours. The contractions were coming so close together, there was almost no break at all. Doris turned down the lights and left the room to take care of some paperwork, Bruce went down to admitting, and Heather stayed with me.

*Sharon began to slide to a low point—crying some, feeling angry, but still hanging in. I practiced some therapeutic touch as she stood alone in the bathroom doorway.*

*Sharon talked to me about her frustrations at this point and began to relax her mood. I suggested she lie down, hoping she would get her long-awaited break between contractions. Sharon lay on her side; I covered her and held her hand. Two or three minutes passed without a contraction. Bruce arrived with a coffee and muffin. I gestured quietly that I thought Sharon might actually be asleep. I motioned him over to take my place.*

#### 10:00 A.M.

After a few minutes of very welcome sleep, I woke up feeling much better emotionally. Bruce, with coaching from Heather and Doris, stayed with me through each contraction. It was tough needing him and yet being unable to tell him so. Needing him close, and yet so afraid that his touch would set off another painful set of contractions. All I could do was hold tight to his hands and look deeply into his eyes as he tried to help me.

I felt the depth of her pain, as much as someone outside could sense it, and was overwhelmed by it. I have never experienced pain that was that severe or constant. I knew she could not go back, and that Sharon would want at the end to have not taken any medication. I could see the fear and resistance to each new contraction as it began to build, usually just as the previous one was ending.

At this point I was barely making it through each contraction. Without the support of Bruce, Heather, and Doris, I would have definitely asked for pain medication. But they kept telling me I was doing fine, even though I was sure I was somehow "failing" some sort of labor test. Each contraction I thought, "This is it; I can't take it anymore." Each time a new contraction started before the last had finished I'd cry out "No!" in a loud voice, not caring who heard me. I just wanted the pain to stop. And each time one of them would calmly work with me coaxing, cajoling, demanding, until I would look them in the eye one more time and try to match my breathing with theirs.

Doris, our nurse, was particularly effective at getting Sharon to pant and breath through the peaks as the pain intensified. She, Heather, and I took turns working with Sharon. I was thankful they were there as I found it so hard to see Sharon in such torment that I would lose my focus, which messed up the breathing. Having a caring and skilled team of coaches was critical to me, and I believe to Sharon, to get through this.

Sharon's courage and sheer will to get through each contraction was amazing. She yelled, pleaded, and sometimes asked to "go home now." Mostly she worked with whoever was the coach. She forced herself to breathe, pant, and blow out each breath as one contraction wave rolled through on top of the last.

We tried various positions leaning on the bed, leaning over the bed, lying down, but I found that, for me, I was most comfortable standing. It was really difficult. Standing was tiring me out, but changing positions intensified the contractions to the point where I couldn't stand them. A few times I found myself actually falling asleep standing up during the few seconds between contractions. Heather and Bruce were always there, holding my hands and holding me up when I needed it.

11:00 A.M.

Doris suggested it was time to do a vaginal exam since the urge to push was beginning to become overwhelming. It was hard to get on the bed, but I made it, hoping for news that the baby would be arriving soon. The exam showed that while fully effaced, I was still only 9 centimeters dilated. I was shocked. How could I go to 6 centimeters so fast and then take so long for the next 3? If I was feeling the urge to push I should be fully dilated, shouldn't I? Doris told me it was very important that I not push until that last centimeter had dilated.

I was angry, though I didn't know who to be angry at. This was not what I had been expecting; none of the books or videos or birth stories had prepared me for five hours of almost continuous pain. I needed all the support Bruce could give me at this point and, again, he was right there for me.

The next hour was very difficult. I worked with Sharon a lot at this point. As we stood, hands clenched, I felt that we were in some bizarre ritualistic dance. Our eyes locked together, our arms moving up and around, our breathing in unison. It was extremely intimate as we breathed through the contractions one at a time. It was a moving meditation, with our short intense breathing our mantra.

At one point, I reminded Sharon that the only way out was through. We had no choice but to work through each contraction. I was concerned that she might direct her anger at me, but she seemed to understand and focused even more on getting through the contractions.

## 12:00 NOON

By noon I was getting desperate and was losing the struggle to resist pushing. Everyone was getting stressed. Dr. Sheppard had returned and did another exam, finding that the cervix still had about half a centimeter to go. I couldn't believe it. How could the cervix still not be open after the last hour? The doctor suggested rupturing my membranes, which surprisingly were still intact at this point. I had refused the first time the nurse had suggested rupturing, wanting the birth to be as natural as possible, but now was willing to try it. Once again, I felt I was at the end of my rope, and once again, Heather was right there for me.

*I further explained that standing might help put more pressure on the cervix and thus increase the progress. The next half hour was very hard for Sharon. The nurse set a goal of half an hour before the next internal exam in order to minimize the number of exams done on Sharon. The intensity of interaction between Sharon and Bruce during this last hour was marvelous to witness. Their focus into each other's eyes, whether standing, kneeling over the back of the bed, or holding both hands never wavered. I'm sure I saw Sharon deepen and age. Her face changed and the concentration revealed an older, even more confident woman. Bruce had been unflappable throughout, ever vigilant and supportive.*

The urge to push became impossible to resist. Each contraction I could feel it getting stronger and stronger. They would all try so hard to get me to pant to prevent the pushing, but I kept crying out "I can't!" as my body dropped automatically into a semi-squat position, and they would say "You can," and then one of them would capture my eyes and help me to stand, and lead me through the panting one more time. Doris was particularly effective at this point. Her mesmerizing light blue eyes and quiet voice could get through to me when nothing else could.

12:30 P.M.

Finally at 12:30, I had my last exam. This one revealed that the baby had already started her descent down the birth canal. Even though that final stubborn lip of the cervix was still there: Dr. Sheppard actually had to push it out of the way. This time there was no holding back—the baby was coming!

Dr. Sheppard suddenly remembered the cord blood kit, and she and Doris scrambled to get it ready while Heather and Bruce helped me get into position on the birthing bed. Heather coached me to refine my position and think of the direction my body needed to be in to push. I remembered reading in my Feldenkrais birthing book how to tuck under my tailbone to make a smooth channel for the baby to come through. Heather had me draw up my knees and she took one leg while Bruce took the other.

Fortunately Dr. Sheppard was ready because I couldn't hold back the pushing any longer. It felt so wonderful to finally be allowed to do what my body had been aching to do for the past hour and a half. Suddenly I wasn't tired anymore. I felt a rush of energy, and I let out a few very loud groans with the first pushes that helped release some of the pent-up frustration.

Then, the doctor began giving me instructions on how she wanted the pushing done, to help the baby and to minimize the damage to my perineum. Finally, I felt like I was doing something right. I found I had complete control of my pushing-muscles and could do whatever pushing was needed. It didn't even seem to matter if there was a contraction or not.

Everything that had gone before seemed to be leading up to this moment in time. All the horse riding I had done during the pregnancy to keep muscles in tone, all the Shiatsu treatments to learn to release tense muscles, all the bottled-up urge to push, and most of all, the fact that I had made it this far without drugs, so I had full sensation where I needed it.

*The coordination between Sharon's short effective pushes and Dr. Sheppard's quiet and soft instructions—"push again," "now ease up," "now push," "stop and blow a little"—produced a gentle pushing stage until the baby's head slowly emerged.*

12:28 P.M.
I was so glad that Bruce was there with me. That he was sharing this moment when the baby arrived.

Suddenly, I could see the top of our daughter's head. A reddish blue shape. With each push instruction, the doctor would gently move the perineum back and around the emerging head. It was amazing. Our little girl was being born. This happened quickly as the head came through and then the chest.

Suddenly, the mood of the doctor seemed to change. She had asked if Bruce wanted to cut the cord, but now, with the baby still only half out, she asked Doris for the scissors so she could cut the cord herself.

*With grace and concentration, Dr. Sheppard slid her fingers between the baby's neck and the cord, which was tightly wrapped around her neck. She clipped it, cut it, and nodded to Sharon to push hard to birth the body quickly. Sharon did this with ease, and the rather limp baby was whisked over for a rubdown and extra oxygen.*

The medical team all went with the baby, leaving Bruce and me on our own, not knowing what was wrong.

I had wanted to hand the baby to Sharon, but Dr. Sheppard just looked at me and shook her head. In an instant, an OB and pediatrician had come in and with Dr. Sheppard and Doris were standing and working with the baby.

I felt a sudden alarm go off and realized that something was wrong. How wrong I didn't know. I heard Doris say that she had a heartbeat, which reassured me. At one point the baby rolled its head sideways and looked directly at Sharon; she seemed to know Sharon. Again it was amazing.

If it hadn't been for Heather standing right beside me and telling me exactly what was going on, I think I would have panicked. She told me the cord had been wrapped around the baby, so they had to cut it before she was born, but the baby had a heartbeat and they were giving her oxygen. She told me the baby was breathing. She told me she could see the baby moving.

*I explained to Sharon what was happening and why the baby needed almost everyone's attention. We listened as Sharon whispered, "Breathe, baby, breathe." The baby's heartbeat was strong, and after four anxious minutes, we heard her muffled cry behind the oxygen mask. The baby's APGAR score jumped from 2 to 7 in five minutes of being born. A pediatrician provided reassurance that all was well, and the new baby girl was lifted from the warming unit onto Sharon's chest. We unwrapped her, and Sharon hugged her baby, skin to skin, and Bruce hugged Sharon.*

We could finally be with our daughter. She was so tiny and perfectly formed. Truly a miracle. We mostly stared at each other. I felt a huge sense of love for Sharon and the baby and breathed a huge sigh of relief.

It was incredible holding her warm body next to mine, feeling her small movements as she nestled close, hearing her breathe. I wanted to hold her, and to hold Bruce, all at the same time. She was okay; my wonderful baby girl was just fine.

With the sense of relief that the baby was here and all was well came another relief—the ordeal was finally over—the painful contractions had stopped. I could feel my body trembling with relief. Nothing had ever felt so good as simply not feeling the pain anymore.

*At 2 minutes to 1 P.M., not only a baby was born, but we witnessed the birth of a mother and the start of a new family.*

1:10 P.M.
Once the baby was okay, Dr. Sheppard came back and drew the blood needed for the cord blood kit, helped me birth the placenta, stitched one small tear, and then said goodbye. Bruce got out the video camera and captured some of those first few precious moments on film. Then he took a still picture of Heather and me and the new baby.

Heather stayed for another half hour or so. She helped me try to feed the baby, but the baby seemed more interested in looking around than eating, though she did give my breast a few licks and seemed to like the taste of colostrum.

When Heather left, Bruce and I were alone with our new daughter for the first time. We talked about the experience we'd just shared, we hugged each other close, but mostly, we just marveled at the tiny miracle that was now in our care.

# To Tell a Birth Story . . .

Women have been telling birth stories since the beginning of time. In the Bible, many people's names are based on their birth or conception experience. For example, Sara's son was named Isaac, or *Yitzchak* in Hebrew. *Yitzchak* means "will laugh," referring to the joy of Abraham and Sara after years of infertility.

For me, talking about the birth of my sons served as a healing experience after the birth of my first son, Menachem, and as a way of reliving the experience after the birth of my son, Eliezer. I also kept a box with the hospital name tags, measuring tape and other odds and ends, like the pen and pad from the hospital. This is my way of preserving the memories of their births.

Here are few ways that you can preserve your child's birth:

**Write as you experience your birth.** Keep a running journal as you go into labor, until you can no longer concentrate (or remember!) to write down your feelings and thoughts. You can fill in the details at the end after the birth.

**Record your birth story on tape.** It's not always easy to get your thoughts down on paper. If you find it easier to talk about your birth, then try recording your birth story on tape. Choose a quiet day when you will not be interrupted, perhaps a day that your partner can take the baby for a walk. If you find yourself at a loss for words, pretend that you are talking to your best friend. Tell her all the details, everything you thought, everything you felt. Don't be shy! If you don't like what you recorded, you can always go back and erase it.

**Draw or paint a representation of the birth.** Borrow the book *Birthing from Within* by Pam England for inspiration and ideas on birth art. There are many examples of real women's drawings, and their thoughts behind the drawings.

**Make a memory box.** You can use any box: a shoebox or a nicer wooden or plastic box. Inside, place all the name tags, first photos of the baby, registration paper, photocopies of the birth certificate, and so on. You can also include the recording of your birth story, or artwork, or written birth story. Hide in a safe place, and take it out to cherish on special days.

# PART THREE

# The Postpartum Doula

# CHAPTER 9

# Meeting the Needs of New Mothers

I REMEMBER THE FIRST days and weeks after my first son's birth. I read several baby care books, trying to reconcile the barrage of conflicting advice I was receiving. Is my baby getting enough milk? Is breastfeeding supposed to hurt? Should I wake my baby up to nurse? Do all babies cry this much? I had so many questions.

"Sleep when the baby sleeps," was the most common bit of advice I received, but when exactly was I supposed to sleep?! Friends and family were visiting throughout the day, and there was so much to do: laundry to wash and fold, meals to cook, baby clothes to organize. And even if I could sleep when my baby slept, when should I eat? And how could I shower?

A labor doula provides minimal post-labor support, unless she also offers postpartum doula services. Your need for support does not end after birth. If you compare becoming a parent to moving to a new country, the labor doula helps you travel over the ocean, and a postpartum doula acts as your tour guide, advocate, and interpreter for your first few weeks. The postpartum doula helps you find answers to your questions; cares for your new baby and you; empowers you to discover and stand up for your parenting ideals; and helps with older siblings, light housekeeping, and cooking.

# What New Mothers Need Most

What I needed help with most after my second child was much the same as with my first. I still had questions, I worried just as much, and I was actually even more tired, considering I now had a toddler to chase after!

Whether you are having your first or third child, you'll find yourself with questions and needs. Postpartum doulas provide support in four general areas: baby feeding support, baby care, mother care, and home management.

## BABY FEEDING SUPPORT

Whether you decide to breastfeed or formula feed, you'll have many questions and support needs, both practical and emotional.

> "I think a postpartum doula is more important than a birth doula. During birth, it's the mom who has to do all the work. Postpartum, the doula can take care of household chores, watch other children, and provide tangible assistance that makes such a big difference for the new mom."
> —Jennifer, California

If you're breastfeeding, you may feel embarrassed if things don't go smoothly, wondering how something so natural could be so confusing. You may wonder if you're the only mother who feels pain during nursing—especially when so many breastfeeding books say that breastfeeding should not hurt. You may worry that your baby is not getting enough milk, or you could be contending with a premature or jaundiced infant. A postpartum doula can help with all these concerns, answer questions, and refer you to a lactation consultant or medical professional, if the situation warrants expert help.

If you cannot breastfeed or choose to formula feed, you may have as many questions as a breastfeeding mother. What kind of

> **☙ A MOTHERING MOMENT . . .**
>
> "I couldn't believe the hospital let me take home this fragile little newborn after only giving me brief instructions on how to diaper, breastfeed, etc. I was so frightened. Esther taught me the basics in baby care but also gave me confidence that I had good mommy instincts and that I was doing a great job. I needed that."
> —Claire, Michigan

equipment do you need? How should the bottles be prepared? Is there a preferred way to hold the baby while feeding her? Do you need to sterilize the bottles and nipples—and if yes, how?

## BABY CARE

Changing a diaper seemed so easy—until I had my own little one! I was worried about his umbilical stump being rubbed, and my son's diapers always leaked. Plus, I made quite a few calls to the doctor to ask about some sniffling and strange breathing sounds my baby was making. (Turned out to be normal, thank God.)

And I'll never forget my son's first bath. My husband and I laid out all the paraphernalia, closely following the step-by-step instructions from a baby care book. My husband wanted to make sure the baby shampoo was safe, so he rubbed the soap into his own eyes!

Now, I look back and laugh at how nervous and cautious we were, but when you're a first time parent, no matter how many kids you've cared for as a babysitter, you can't help but be overwhelmed.

Postpartum doulas don't just answer questions, but actually show you how to care for your newborn. She's not there to hold the baby while you clean the house, though she'll certainly help with the baby if you want to rest, eat, or shower. The postpartum doula's goal is to help you feel confident in caring for your baby.

Second-time parents often have as many questions as first-time mothers. My second son's temperament was very different from my first, so everything I knew about calming a baby seemed not to work! Plus, my second son was slightly jaundiced, and I was always worried that I wasn't knowledgeable enough to know when to call the doctor. But the most difficult part of becoming a mom for the second time was learning how to care for a toddler and a newborn at the same time. A doula's education and experience enables her to answer questions like these.

### MOTHER SUPPORT

Family and friends tend to focus on the baby and ignore your needs as a new mother. This is entirely normal—they're excited to meet this new little person, but they've known you for years. The postpartum doula's number one priority is you. How are you coping with motherhood? How are you feeling after the birth? The doula will help cook healthful meals and bring you water to drink whenever you sit down to nurse the baby. (It's easy to forget about your health when caring for a newborn!)

"Nurturing the mother means 'mothering' [her] so she can mother her own baby," says Vicky York, a certified postpartum doula who has worked with over 600 families. "It means helping her with whatever is holding her up from taking care of her baby with confidence, strength, and joy. It may mean cooking for her, listening to her, watching the baby so she can sleep, finding resources for her, cleaning her house, teaching her how to bathe the baby, or clipping his nails. I once had to plant 90 zinnias on a hot day because if I didn't do it, the mom would have done it to prepare for out-of-town guests whom she wanted to impress with her zinnia bed."

You'll most likely have questions about your personal health, perhaps questions you would feel embarrassed to ask your doctor,

### 🐾 A MOTHERING MOMENT . . .

"After my c-section, everyone told me to take it easy, not to walk around much, and avoid climbing steps. After about six days of following this cautious advice, I was longing to go outside. It was a beautiful spring day, and I wanted to take a walk around the neighborhood. Leslie showed me how to use the sling and offered me reassurance that the baby was safe and comfortable in there. She walked with me around the neighborhood, adjusting her pace to match mine. The walk really lifted my spirits, and without Leslie, I would not have had the energy or confidence to do it." —Rebecca, Pennsylvania

midwife, or a friend. How much bleeding is normal? When will it stop? Is the cramping you feel considered normal? How soon can you be intimate with your partner, and what can you expect from those romantic moments post-birth?

If you experience a difficult delivery, either a cesarean section or any other physically damaging birth, a postpartum doula will be key to helping you heal faster. You may not be able to go up and down stairs more than once a day, so simple household chores and caring for older children will not be easy. Also, carrying the baby or getting out of bed may be painful. Breastfeeding may also seem more complicated if you can't lay the baby on your stomach. A doula can show you how to care for your little one without causing pain to yourself. Plus, she'll explain how to care for your stitches and show you how to get in and out of bed with the least amount of pain and breastfeed without the baby pressing on your tender abdomen.

The postpartum doula's role is particularly essential if you experience a traumatic birth. "It may help you to discuss it with someone who understands the birth process and may have worked with other

"On days when the doula did not come to my house, I literally watched the clock all day till it was time for my husband to come home. When he arrived at the front door, I typically burst into tears the minute I saw him and handed our baby to him so that I could have a few moments to myself. On days that the doula had been at our house, my husband would arrive home to find that dinner was ready, the dishes were done, and I was usually relaxing on the couch with the baby, and we were both calm and happy. The experience of having someone come and take care of me during the day was wonderful, and in turn, I didn't have as many demands from my husband, who was also overwhelmed from working all day and then immediately being faced with a war zone when he entered the house." —Laura, Oregon

women in similar circumstances," says Marlene Gubler, a postpartum doula in Pennsylvania. "Depending on the experience, I may even suggest a support group or have her call another client with a similar birth, who is willing to talk things over with her. I am always available to my clients, 24 hours a day and 7 days a week, to talk through the birth process. Some moms need their feelings validated, and some moms need to know they can voice their feelings without being judged."

While a doula cannot provide psychological or medical help from a professional standpoint, she can listen to your thoughts and fears. Vicky York explains, "Some women just want me to listen while they describe what they didn't get in terms of mothering from their own mothers, or their childhood sexual abuse, or their fears about inadequacy in childrearing, or anything."

## HOME MANAGEMENT

The baby just woke from his 10-minute nap and wants to nurse, and you may be exhausted. If that wasn't enough, laundry is piling up, dishes have been sitting for days, and you don't even know what you're making for dinner! A postpartum doula can help with the laundry, keep the dishes and kitchen under control, and help with cooking and meal planning.

While it's nice to think that visiting family, older children, or your partner will be able to help around the house, usually it does not work out that way. Having a doula who can help keep the house together during the first few weeks can relieve so much stress.

# Lactation Consultants, Baby Nurses, Maids, and Doulas: What's the Difference?

You may be wondering what's the difference between a postpartum doula and a lactation consultant? Or a maid? Or a babysitter? The most significant difference is their training and ultimate goals. A lactation consultant is there to help you with any breastfeeding problems. A maid's main goal is to clean your house, and a babysitter is there to watch the kids. A doula is there for you, and she will help with whatever you need most that day.

Here are more details on how services provided by maids, babysitters, baby nurses, and lactation consultants differ from postpartum doula support.

## BABY NURSES

Both doulas and baby nurses help care for the baby, but a baby nurse does not provide mother care, help with housework, or provide any other services that are not directly related to the newborn. Usually, a baby nurse works in 24-hour shifts and may live in your home for an extended period of time, sometimes up to six months. The services offered are like those of a nanny.

Some baby nurses may tend to take over care of your newborn and are not always keen on educating or empowering you to parent your child. However, when a baby is extremely ill or requires special care, a baby nurse may be necessary. If this is your situation, hire a baby nurse who is willing to teach you how to care for the baby's special needs.

## LACTATION CONSULTANTS

While some postpartum doulas are lactation consultants, not all doulas are certified or educated to treat special problems or breast-feeding challenges. A postpartum doula can answer your basic questions regarding breastfeeding, like positioning and latching the baby properly or making sure the baby is getting enough milk. Postpartum doulas also know how to handle a variety of minor concerns, like cracked and bleeding nipples or waking a sleepy baby to eat.

But there are some special cases when a lactation consultant is needed. When a baby has special needs, like Down's syndrome or cleft palette, or if the baby is premature, a lactation consultant's expertise may be needed. If you have inverted nipples or are experiencing an unusual amount of pain while nursing, a lactation consultant can help.

A postpartum doula is trained to watch you and your baby for warning signs of a problem and will tell you if she thinks medical or expert advice is needed. If you are concerned, she can give references. She may work closely with a lactation consultant, or she may give you numbers of different organizations to help you find a medical expert.

## MAIDS

A postpartum doula really isn't there to scrub your floors. They usually help with the housework you would have done if no one was

"I sought a postpartum doula because of my terror of repeating the recovery from my first birth. I worked very hard towards a VBAC and ended up with another c-section. Deanne changed diapers, rocked the baby, and helped me position him for nursing during the first week when I was still very sore from the surgery. She helped keep me from doing things, like carry anything or walking too much, which would cause more harm than good."
— Shereen, Washington

there to do it for you, like the laundry, dishes, and cleaning up the kitchen. Plus, while the doula is working around the house, she may listen to your concerns and questions, so while she's folding the laundry, you and she may talk about your baby's birth, family concerns, baby care or personal care questions, or whatever is on your mind.

There are times when you need a maid's services. Perhaps you have a large family and need the extra help, or maybe you just don't like to clean. Maybe your mother-in-law tests your bookshelves for dust with white gloves at every visit, and she's coming to see the new baby! Certainly, you may hire a maid to help you prepare your house for the "inspection."

## BABYSITTERS

Usually, you would not hire a babysitter to help with a newborn, but you may hire a babysitter to watch your older children if, for example, you need to bring the baby or yourself to a doctor appointment. A postpartum doula helps with older children, but usually she's not just watching the kids.

As mentioned before, a postpartum doula can help take over some of your normal day-to-day tasks that you're just not ready to handle right now. She may take the kids to the park while you rest with the baby or help transport the older kids to and from friends' homes or activities. A postpartum doula may come in the morning to help get the children ready for school or may encourage and teach older children to care for their baby sister or brother. She may also help the children accept their new baby brother or sister and can also help you adjust to caring for an additional child.

## CHAPTER 10

# Comfort Measures and Services a Postpartum Doula Provides

THE SERVICES THAT POSTPARTUM doulas offer differ from client to client. You may be looking for someone to help you with parenting and breastfeeding, but you have family to help you with cooking and housework. Perhaps this is your fourth child, and you're looking for help with your older children and want someone to take care of you, for a change! You most likely have a general idea of why you'd like to hire a postpartum doula, but even so, take some notes while reading this chapter. Mark down what you think you'd like from your doula, so you can compare your expectations with her services and help her nurture you and your family.

Like labor doulas, postpartum doulas provide informational, emotional, physical, and practical support. Let's take a closer look at the way they do this.

## Informational Support

In the 1970s, writer Dana Raphael coined the word "doula" in her book, *The Tender Gift*, to describe a woman who helped the new mother physically and emotionally during the postpartum period,

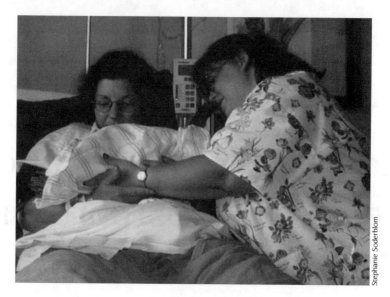

FIGURE 10.1 Doula Stephanie Soderblom helps a mother
position her newborn to breastfeed.

encouraging a successful breastfeeding relationship between mother
and child.

## BREASTFEEDING

"I help a mother with breastfeeding by (hopefully) being there when
the baby is born and helping with that initial contact right after
birth," says Michelle Cousins, a postpartum doula from Virginia. "I
do use a hands-on approach whenever necessary. Sometimes you
have to help the mother adjust her breast to bring the baby to it and
to show how to unlatch. I have never had a mother mind the hands-
on approach, as there really isn't any other way to help.

"I encourage breastfeeding often (let the baby be your cue), and I
encourage the mother to talk and look at her baby while feeding,"
continues Cousins. "I also tell her about the color, amount, and tex-
ture of diapers from breastfed babies . . . how to tell the difference between diarrhea and [normal]. If her nipples are sore, lanolin helps

greatly, and the baby can still nurse after application. Also, applying a little breast milk after a feeding can help sore or tender nipples."

Every doula's approach to breastfeeding support is different, depending on her training and personality. Whether you need more hands-on help, or prefer a more distant approach, let your doula know. "One thing that is unique about me is that I am a low-touch doula," says Kimberly Bepler, a postpartum doula from Oregon. "I often have clients who are low- to no-touch. While they are breastfeeding, I will arrange pillows for their utmost comfort, and I bring food and drinks to nourish them. However, I do not invade their private space unless requested to, or to facilitate with breastfeeding in the early days."

One of the most common concerns with regard to breastfeeding is whether the baby is getting enough milk. "[The worry] may come directly from the first-time mom, or it could have been suggested by one of the grandmothers who did not breastfeed her children," says Barbara J. Coscia, a postpartum doula from Connecticut, and owner and founder of Mother to Mother. "Many discussions take place to reassure the new mom that she is on the right track and everything is working fine."

The doula can also help with practical questions. "I tell [my clients] to buy large button-up shirts which make it easy for nursing, and 'busy' prints hide leaks," says Cousins. "I also tell them to try different bras and see which nursing bras they are able to unhook one-handed and re-hook the same way. The more you practice at it, the better you get! I also

> "Denise was invaluable, helping me with latch-on and different nursing positions. She also helped me master the breast pump, with which I had problems at first. She was encouraging and respectful of my feelings and frustration." —Jennifer, California

advise bringing a cloth diaper or a receiving blanket to help you feel more discrete, especially if nursing in public. I tell them it is not against the law to nurse in public and to not feel ashamed to do so. They should never feel that they have to go into a bathroom stall to feed their baby."

A doula is also trained to look out for situations that warrant outside help, either from a doctor or lactation consultant. If a special situation arises, your doula can provide you with relevant contact information. Some doulas are lactation consultants, while others may have personal experience breastfeeding and look to their training and experience to help you.

"She was supportive and provided books for me to borrow, a breastfeeding pillow to try. She also bought me a couple of nursing bras after my milk came in. The ones I had purchased were way too small." —Jennifer, California

"I had a client with twins who decided to breastfeed and wasn't sure how to get the babies to latch on at the same time," tells Marlene Gubler, a postpartum doula from Pennsylvania. "She was much like a deer in the headlights the first time we did it. I think she was a bit surprised when I guided her and just started positioning everyone together, but, as the days went on, she needed less and less guidance with getting the boys latched. I knew my time was almost done there when I walked in the door one morning, and there sat mom, with both boys latched and a huge smile on her face. She was so full of pride and self-confidence as a mom. It was quite rewarding to see such a moment."

## FORMULA FEEDING

If you're formula feeding, a doula can help you with the practicalities. "I make sure they know how to clean bottles, make formula properly, and feed the baby," says doula Crystal Sada. "I also en-

### ❧ A MOTHERING MOMENT . . .

"Perhaps the most striking memories following the birth of my son are those involving early tandem nursing experiences. My daughter was 2½ at the time and feeling excited yet somewhat unsure of the new baby. Our first time as a triad instead of dyad was in the delivery room when my son refused to nurse right away. Big sister was very proud that she could 'teach' him how to nurse. The response of the observing medical workers was of course shock and some discomfort, but he finally latched on and I held both of them together, she gently touching his face while the two of them suckled. My doula was priceless at this point as she sheltered us from the business around us and gave us those precious few moments 'alone.'" —Bianca, Ohio

courage them to always hold the baby for feeding so that the bonding takes place, and remind them to switch the sides they feed the baby on, so the baby is stimulated from both angles, just like a breastfed baby would be."

Both breastfeeding and formula feeding moms deal with engorged breasts and may need to treat clogged milk ducts. A doula can suggest different ways to reduce discomfort. Depending on your circumstances, your doula may suggest taking warm showers, placing cabbage leaves inside your bra against your breasts, or massaging the breast in a particular way to encourage a clogged milk duct to loosen, or a variety of other tips and tricks.

### BABY CARE AND PARENTING

You may have questions on colic, calming a crying baby, treating diaper rash, or watching for jaundice. Or you may want someone

"Denise helped us create a list of the items that we would need for baby's hygiene and care, which included ointments, powders, washes, medicines, clippers, etcetera. She recommended a couple of toys, and some items we had missed. Once baby was home, she showed us how to diaper, trim nails, and easily bathe the baby. She showed us different carrying positions to help soothe her when she was colicky or just fussy. She helped us figure out what to dress her in, and how to swaddle her." —Jennifer, California

nearby when you give your baby a bath or change the baby's diaper, just to feel more confident that you're doing things correctly. Your doula is there to help you feel more confident in caring for your baby.

Your doula may help you find your parenting style. There are so many "methods" and approaches, and few mothers strictly follow one approach. Your doula may lend you books to read, videos to watch, or provide copies of articles or research papers.

"I provide my clients with informational support through an extensive lending library, pamphlets, and other written forms from various sources," says Cousins. "Many of my sources are other groups such as La Leche League, Bradley classes, and midwifery and doula groups. Some information comes from chiropractors and herbalists. Some information is available through medical groups and even some from the Internet."

While your doula may have strong feelings on parenting philosophies, her job is not to tell you what to do or not do with your family. A professional doula's goal is to empower you to feel more confident as a mother and to help you find resources, so you can make your own choices.

"I try to remember that all of us are different, have different philosophies, religions, and ways of handling life," says postpartum doula Karen Schroeder, owner of Embracing Birth. "Parenting is the same thing. There is no book; it's by trial and error, so let the new parents learn as they go. I try to guide them with as much information as they ask for. Ultimately the choices they make, right or wrong, are theirs."

"When a mother or father asks me, 'What would you do?' I try and turn it around and say 'Well, what are your instincts telling you to do?' It is in that empowerment that great parents are developed," explains doula Crystal Sada. "So to me it is always about empowering the parents to make their own wise decisions for their family, and I do not cross that line. . . . I just provide valid information and sit back and guide them."

# Emotional Support

After the birth of my second son, I felt as if I was floating. I was happy and eager to start mothering my new baby. I had a beautiful birth and was constantly replaying the scenes in my mind. I wanted so much to share my birth story with someone, but really had no one who would appreciate the details that I wanted to express.

Family from out of town was coming, which went against my instinct to hide away from the world and just concentrate on me and my immediate family. While I wanted to see my relatives, as we live miles apart, I felt overwhelmed knowing I had

"My doulas were a positive force. They made me feel as if I was doing a great job as a mother, and to have that confidence was very reassuring, especially in such an isolating culture as New York."
—Jennifer, New York

to entertain and cook for everyone, when all I wanted to do was sleep and nurse. Whenever I started thinking about all the people and everything I had to do, I would start crying, sometimes out of the blue. I wasn't even that upset; I just could not help it! Baby blues struck, and what I wanted most was someone to talk to who would acknowledge my feelings and understand.

A postpartum doula will be there to listen to your thoughts and feelings. She'll let you tell your birth story over and over, and she won't judge you.

"Mothers can become overwhelmed with emotion, as they experience changing levels of progesterone and estrogen, coping with the physical discomforts of giving birth, breast discomfort, fatigue, and trying to keep it all together while the doorbell buzzes, the telephone rings, and throngs of well-wishers are dropping by to see the new baby," explains doula Karen Schroeder. "Luckily, it doesn't last forever. A good venting of your feelings and a good cry can bring relief and help to chase those blues away. The important thing to remember is that the 'baby blues' are temporary, and usually by the second week, you begin to feel better physically and emotionally."

> "I felt alone and overwhelmed, and Leslie kept me company. She assured me that I was doing fine with the baby and that it was okay to feel a little bit down."—Rebecca, Pennsylvania

Dealing with family during the postpartum period can be especially draining. Even if you usually get along with family, your delicate emotional state can make "innocent" comments or unsolicited advice from family or friends seem like declarations of war! Your doula can help buffer family confrontations, and may even help educate them on your needs.

"Sometimes I have to be the 'heavy' and turn guests away because mom and baby need rest," explains Cousins. "I have had to

"It had been a particularly difficult and tiring day (and night before) with my newborn son. I was stressed out and desperately tired, and I knew the next day was going to be a big one, in which a lot of family and friends were gathering for a religious ceremony for the baby. I got a call from two elder relatives who said they couldn't wait until the next day and were coming over that night, within the hour, to meet the baby! My house was not exactly neat as a pin, and I was in no state to entertain.

"My postpartum doula was great! She made sure I put a very cute outfit on the baby and then eat something and find a snack for the visiting relatives. She watched the baby while I made myself presentable. And she convinced me that my family would not even notice the messy house—only the baby. Of course she was right! Because she helped me pull things (and myself!) together, I actually enjoyed the visit!" —Rivka, New York

nicely talk to mothers and mothers-in-law about how they talk to the new mom and how they need to give the mom some space. I have never had anyone get angry at me, at least not yet. But the mother is my 'mother' and I am there to protect her and do what she wants me to do. If that means telling the mother-in-law to take a walk, well, so be it."

## "BABY BLUES"

Many women, as much as 80 percent, experience some postpartum sadness, usually referred to as the "baby blues." But how do you know if what you're feeling goes beyond the baby blues? According to Depression After Delivery Inc., as many as 1 in 10 women experience postpartum depression. Depression does not just go away with time. Talking with other mothers or with a clinical psychologist, or taking medications may help.

Dr. Wendy Newhouse Davis, a counselor, consultant, and founder of Baby Blues Connection (a mom-to-mom support group in Oregon), answers some questions on postpartum depression.

Q. **What's the difference between baby blues and postpartum depression?**

A. "It is estimated that up to 80 percent of all moms will have the 'baby blues,' which is marked by symptoms such as mood swings, irritability, anxiety, and crying jags. This is a transitory condition that occurs within the first week or two postpartum, and is improved by rest, support, good nutrition, and time.

"In contrast, postpartum depression has many of the same symptoms but rather than beginning to feel better, mom feels worse and starts to feel overwhelmed and hopeless. Not every woman who has these early symptoms will end up with a true postpartum depression, but any distress in adjustment will be helped by reaching out and getting more support. If she does have postpartum depression, reaching out early will make a significant difference in her recovery.

"Twenty percent of all women experience some depression or anxiety in the postpartum year. Sometimes anxiety and depression merge with the early baby blues, but the onset might be any time in the first year. She might have one or more of these symptoms: sadness, crying, fear, numb emotions, irritability, anger, confusion, insomnia, or obsessive thoughts. Sometimes women experience these symptoms after rapid weaning, when periods resume, or after going on hormonal birth control."

Q. **When should a mother seek help?**

A. "If she is feeling distress, difficulty with her moods or thoughts, insomnia or irritability that lasts longer than two weeks, it is important that she reach out to a knowledgeable resource for postpartum adjustment and depression. If she feels down or angry or anxious, it helps to start talking about it (to supportive people) as soon as she feels able. This is true whether she is diagnosed with a postpartum mood disorder or not.

"The symptoms of postpartum depression, anxiety, or obsessive compulsive disorder cause a woman to feel shame and hopelessness at the same time as she is overwhelmed with a new baby and postpartum recovery. The combination of shame and the inability to think clearly make it nearly impossible for her to reach out. Considering that about one in five women will have some depression or anxiety after childbirth, it seems that we should hear more about it. Because people hesitate to talk about it, many women end up feeling embarrassed and scared that they are alone. They are not alone. There are other women to connect with who have recovered from postpartum distress and recovery, and there are professionals, websites, and books that can offer information and reassurance. A woman needs to remember that she will get better, no matter how helpless she might feel at first. Postpartum depression and anxiety are temporary, treatable, and common conditions."

Q. **What help is available?**

A. "She can find local resources and links by contacting these national resources: Postpartum Support International at www.postpartum.net or DAD at www.depressionafterdelivery.com. She does not need to wait for her postpartum checkup to talk to her practitioner, but should call earlier if she is having trouble."

Q. **What can you do for yourself?**

A. "Get educated, and keep reaching out until you find the support you need. It is available and it will help. For relief of difficult symptoms, use remedies that are medical, nutritional, or naturopathic.

Some women treat depression and anxiety with antidepressants or anti-anxiety medication, some with natural remedies, some with diet and exercise, some with emotional support. Some use all of them. Find what works best for you.

"Women often compare themselves negatively to other women or to previous role models, and feel inadequate and hopeless. When you are depressed, your self-esteem suffers and you will see most things through a negative filter, including yourself. It is so important to ease the expectations we place on ourselves, find our own way of motherhood, learn to honor it, and take care of ourselves."

Q. How can a doula help?

A. "Help mom create and stick to a plan of self-care and support. Share information with partner and family. Help develop goals that can be broken down to very manageable steps. Offer reassurance, encouragement, guidance to resources, and of course lighten the load at home so mom can tend to herself."

Caring for a new baby can be overwhelming, whether you're a new or veteran parent. Even if you're not nervous about the basics of baby care, the to-do list may never seem to deplete. You may be exhausted from lack of sleep, or you may feel physically weak from birth. Your doula's presence and attitude can be healing, helping you feel that you can get through the tough days.

While we are busy caring for our little one, we also want to be nurtured ourselves. Your doula's main goal is to *mother* you, to make you feel special and taken care of. This aspect of emotional support cannot be overemphasized. When you feel taken care of and appreciated, your stress levels go down, you feel more in control, and your risk of postpartum depression naturally declines.

"I usually am a one-woman cheering squad! My nature is to be very enthusiastic, and most of my clients prefer this," explains postpartum doula Kimberly Bepler. "However, I do have some that need more patience and understanding, and then I work to nurture my quiet side! I also try hard to anticipate their needs, and do 'the little things' that help them feel important. I fix comfort food, like scrambled eggs and new potatoes, or change their bedding to keep things looking fluffy and kept up. Sometimes these things can be as nurturing emotionally as a good chat. Mostly I try to make them feel good about the job they are doing and how much their baby loves them."

If you experience a negative birth, having someone to talk to about your feelings and fears is essential. Talking over the details of what went wrong and what went well allows you accept the birth and process the emotions. Your doula will not only empathetically listen, but she also can provide resources for birth counseling services, if you need extra help.

"Our doula helped me become comfortable with taking the baby out of the house. I was so nervous about taking the baby to the store because I was so worried that she would start crying in public, and I wouldn't be able to deal with it. Our doula accompanied me on several excursions, and this helped build my confidence for taking the baby out on my own." —Laura, Oregon

# Physical Support

Even if you had a relatively easy birth, your body is in the process of returning to its pre-pregnancy state. Your uterus is busy contracting to its normal size, your internal organs are settling back into place, and your hormones are flowing in overtime. Many women are surprised by the intensity of afterpains, or the cramps caused by contractions of the uterus as it returns to its normal size. Add in a sore perineum, engorged breasts, aching muscles, and exhaustion, and it's a miracle you find the strength to get up at night with the baby!

Taking the time to recover is a challenge. Your doula can help you find the time to nap and rest. She can watch your older children, by taking them to the park or bringing them to school or extracurricular activities. She may carry the newborn in a sling while she works around the house, so you can take a nap.

### SLEEP AND RELAXATION

Some doulas offer nighttime support, so you can sleep better. "[For nighttime support], I work 8 hours minimum, up to 10, so that I am not driving while nearly asleep," explains postpartum doula Kimberly Bepler. "I sleep when the baby sleeps, except in special situations. Usually I sleep on the couch, or in a guest room, or on the floor in the baby's room. Usually I bottlefeed the baby on demand throughout the night, or bring the baby to mom for a feeding, and then I am the soother until the baby is back to sleep. I won't work more than two nights a week, and it gets very sticky if I have daytime work scheduled as well. I charge more, but I feel it is worth it, and there really is no price on a good night's sleep."

> "She would change the sheets when I wasn't looking and hold Stella while I took a shower or took a nap! Oh, was that glorious!"
> —Joan, Oregon

If you're having a difficult time relaxing, or your muscles are aching, a massage can help. "Massage feels great and can encourage physical, mental, and emotional relaxation for mom," says postpartum doula Marlene Gubler. "You actually use muscles during labor that you never knew you had . . . and your muscles may feel it later. Physical massage can encourage healing by helping distribute excessive fluids and improving circulation, or massage may help realign organs and encourage uterine contractions to expel excess blood and help the uterus get back to its pre-pregnancy size. Mentally and emotionally, massage helps mom feel pampered, supported, and able to face her postpartum period in a positive way. She may feel better with the 4:00 A.M. feeding after she feels some of her needs are met."

Some doulas can demonstrate infant massage. "Massage for newborns is great for circulation, digestion, and the pleasures of touch," explains Gubler. "I teach moms and dads massage techniques to do with their infants."

Sometimes what you need most is the chance to pamper or care for yourself. Your doula can watch the baby so you can take a hot bath or shower. She can prepare hot tea or light some scented candles. Whatever will help you relax and feel good about yourself, she's there to help.

If you experience a difficult birth or a surgery, your doula can show you how to feed your baby or get in and out of bed more comfortably. If you're unable to walk up and down the stairs, your doula can set a comfortable rest spot and diaper-changing station on the first floor.

> "She made sure I got both enough rest and exercise (leisurely walks through the neighborhood). She made sure we ate balanced, nutritious, and delicious meals and helped me with ice packs and medications." —Jennifer, California

**Helpful Hints for Helping Your Baby Sleep.** I have many fond memories of rocking and nursing my newborn late at night. I loved to gently rub his back, to look out the window at the stars, to smell his baby scent, and so on. Even so, I needed my sleep, and if I spent too much time staring up at the night sky, I was truly exhausted the next day.

Some babies resist sleeping in their cribs or staying asleep at night, and other babies have their days and nights mixed up for the first couple of weeks. Here are some ways to get more sleep, both for you and your baby:

🐦 A MOTHERING MOMENT . . .

"Deanne had brought me a book of possible recipes, and I asked to try this soup. I remember feeling groggy from post-surgery meds, or tired from sitting up and trying to do too much, and then Deanne would heat a bowl of this soup for me. She'd take the baby or entertain my four-year-old and tell me to enjoy—the simple act of getting to slowly eat this incredible bowl of soup that would fill me up would make everything right. Suddenly not having slept, nor being able to move about much, nor able to carry the baby through the house or play for long periods with my eldest seemed less overwhelming. Those bowls of soup would help me remember that it all would work out in time and that I just needed to slow down."
—Shereen, Washington

- *Learn to breastfeed while lying down.* Doula Kimberly Bepler explains, "I have found breastfeeding moms who can learn to nurse in the side-lying position can co-sleep with their babies and gain themselves a lot of rest!" First, make sure your bed is safe for a young baby! Remove all big pillows and comforters from your baby's area, and be sure to place the baby between a guardrail and yourself. Lie the baby down on the bed, and then lie down on your side next to the baby. Place your lower arm above the baby's head, and adjust yourself so that your nipple is at the same height as your baby's mouth. Tease your baby's cheek or lips with your finger or breast until he latches on, and pull the baby towards yourself. For your own comfort, you may want to place something behind your back to lean against, to avoid lying stiffly on your side.

- *Move your baby from your warm body to a warm crib.* The shock of the cool crib sheets can wake your sleeping infant. You can place a heating pad in the crib for a few minutes before you plan on transferring your baby, but be sure to remove the heating pad and touch the sheet before placing the baby down.
- *Give your baby clear signals of when it's time for play and when it's time for sleep.* During the daytime, have the baby nap with the lights on and don't make extra efforts to be quiet, unless, of course, you're napping along with your child! At night, keep everything dark. Don't talk and don't play. If you must change the baby's diaper in the middle of the night, do so in dim lights, or if you can, by the moonlight from a window. Eventually, your baby will adjust.
- *When you nap during the day, turn the phone ringer off and place a note on the door for visitors.* You can record your answering machine message to give all the common answers to the typical questions: "You've reached 555-1212. We're resting with our new baby girl right now. She was born December 5th at 3:35 A.M., and weighed 7 pounds 2 ounces. Mommy and baby are doing fine. If you'd like, please leave a message and we'll get back to you as soon as we can."

## POSTPARTUM NUTRITION

Good nutrition is important during the postpartum period, perhaps even more important than during pregnancy. If you're breastfeeding, your calorie requirements are higher than when you were pregnant. Plus, your body is recovering from childbirth. You need to eat well and keep yourself hydrated, yet you may not have the time or patience to prepare (then sit down for) a balanced meal.

Your doula can help by answering your questions on postpartum nutrition, sharing ideas on healthful snacks and easy meals, and cooking meals for you or your entire family. Your doula can also set up a pitcher of water with cups wherever you spend the most time feeding your baby. Just having someone who will remind you to eat, and then hold the baby while you enjoy your meal, can help!

**Helpful Hints.** Eating right and staying hydrated is not easy when you're a busy and tired mommy. Here are some ways to encourage good eating habits during the postpartum period.

- *Keep a pitcher of water with cups, or a bottle of water, next to your baby-feeding area.* Wherever you choose to nurse or bottlefeed your infant, be sure to have some drinks. This way, every time you feed your infant, you'll have a reminder to drink some water or juice yourself.
- *Have dried fruit and whole wheat crackers available for snacking.* Constipation is a common problem during the postpartum period. Whole grains and fruit can help.
- *Continue taking a prenatal vitamin.* Do this unless otherwise indicated by your caregiver. Just remember that vitamins are supplements, not a replacement, for a well-balanced diet.
- *Include food high in iron.* It's common to have low iron levels after childbirth, and foods high in iron are better than just taking extra iron pills. Examples of foods high in iron are dark leafy greens, beans, and red meat. Try some bean dip with veggies for a snack, or stir-fry pepper steak with rice for dinner.
- *Calcium can be found in a variety of foods, not just dairy products.* Some infants are sensitive to milk and other dairy products. But just because your baby is not able to tolerate milk in your diet doesn't mean you can't get the calcium you need. Almonds and oranges are natural sources, and many juices and breads are fortified with calcium.
- *Forget about losing weight, for now.* If you are breastfeeding, you definitely should not start dieting. But even if you're not

breastfeeding, the immediate postpartum period is not a good time to diet. At least wait until you stop bleeding and you feel generally rested. Then talk to your doctor.

# Practical Support

One thing all mothers need after childbirth is practical help. I personally found that my anxiety levels were the highest when the sink was filled with dirty dishes, the hampers were overflowing, toys were scattered all over the living room, and I had no idea what I was making for dinner. A doula helps with all these common concerns.

"I'm a very practical doula and practice that kind of care for my clients," says doula Kimberly Bepler. "I love to cook and love to just throw things together to please my families. They never know what is in their pantries or fridges, and I laugh every time they say it! I also love to do laundry and folding is one of my favorite household chores. It is also a great thing to do while a mom nurses and I can observe the feeding and encourage her.

"Lesley, stuffed, sealed, and stamped 200 baby announcements that I had pre-addressed. She also helped with the laundry, cooking, and shopping, and general tidying up."
—Jennifer, New York

"I will do light housekeeping, but I tell my clients the deepest scrubbing I do is with a paper towel! Mostly I tidy up, but I will sweep and vacuum, and clean the kitchen. Sometimes I even get to organize the house, starting usually with the baby's room, then I move on to other rooms and closets. This is a fun part of my job, and sometimes gets started by a mom wanting to get rid of her maternity clothes! Sometimes I will run errands with my clients, or at least accompany them out to doctor visits, first day out, and so on.

"I provide whatever the client needs, to the best of my abilities. I will run errands, serve meals to extended family, make calls for products or services, take the baby out for walks in the sling or stroller, give baby baths, even fill the freezer with a month's worth of easy meals. Lately I have wanted to add plant care, since I save more flowers from neglect than your average florist! I also take a lot of photos of baby with mom, since many of these moments happen when no one is around to appreciate them. With clients where I have more hours, I will set the table for a gourmet meal and then take the baby while the new parents enjoy each other."

> "My husband wasn't thrilled about hiring a doula, but once he realized how much it improved our lives, he became her biggest fan!"
> —Laura, Oregon

"[I suggest using] a notebook [where] the family lists what they want done the next day by order of priority for them," explains doula Crystal Sada. "I also ask the couple to sit and talk about what is important to them with the thought in mind that the baby and mother always come first, and if the baby is fussy and the mother is tired, then the laundry may not get done that day. You have to be realistic."

## Family Support

It's not just mothers who can benefit from the services of a postpartum doula.

### FATHERS

Another way doulas provide support is by helping the new father care for the baby. After my first son was born, my husband was nervous about holding or caring for such a tiny baby. He has no younger siblings or cousins, so this truly was a new experience!

Doulas can encourage new fathers to interact with the baby, despite their nervousness.

Your doula can also answer the father's questions and provide ideas on how to help you the most. "I encourage the father to make sure the mother is well-nourished and hydrated, [and suggest] bringing her a drink and pillow when she nurses," says Michelle Cousins, a postpartum doula from Virginia.

But perhaps the most important way doulas help partners is by providing them peace of mind. They know that you and your baby are not alone when they return to work and that you have the help that you deserve and need.

## SIBLINGS

Your doula can also help your older children adjust. "Sometimes we just talk about having a new baby in the house," says Barbara Coscia, owner of Mother to Mother. "We work on finding things that the older child can do to help mommy with the baby, like getting a diaper, baby wipe, or burp cloth so that they feel involved and helpful. Also teaching them to sit on the couch to hold their new brother or sister is a real help to mom and dad."

"I will usually be the siblings' play buddy for a few weeks," says Marlene Gubler. "I once had a little boy, four years old, who was expecting his little brother to come out and start playing ball. He was a bit disappointed that the baby couldn't catch a ball just yet."

> "My husband said simply that the doula provided him peace of mind. Knowing I had someone with me was enough since he couldn't take much time off work."
> —Shereen, Washington

"I will bring projects to work on, and new books they haven't seen before," says Kimberly Bepler. "My favorite is a soap-making project that I can even do with toddlers. I get to be really silly when I have siblings to work with. I make meals, clean up and chase after them, and give their mothers a break for a short time. Some moms hire me to hold their babies while they play with their older child, which is a nice perk of the job!"

## CHAPTER 11

# Hiring a Postpartum Doula

In many areas of the country, there's a shortage of postpartum doulas. With the exception of some large cities, you'll be lucky if you can find five within a thirty-mile radius. To illustrate the point, DoulaWorld.com has twenty labor doulas listed in their database for the state of Massachusetts, but only five are postpartum doulas. Of course, many doulas in Massachusetts are not listed at this Web site, but the ratio between labor and postpartum doulas is clear.

This is why your search should begin early, even if you're still wondering if you want one. Making a few phone calls, and perhaps meeting, may help you decide if you'd like to hire one. Plus, you'll see who's available in your area and have a better idea of how much time you have to make a decision.

"Most doulas can only take on a limited amount of clients at a time," explains Marlene Gubler, a certified doula and Bradley childbirth educator. "If you hire too late, your hours of support may be limited depending on the other clients' needs. I usually tell my clients, first come, first serve. Meaning the first couple to pay a 10 percent deposit of their estimated hours will have their choice of the hours needed. Other potential clients will need to work around those hours. If the first client wants many hours (fifteen to twenty hours per week or more), the next client may only have a choice of every other day and may be limited to two hours per day."

"Currently I have repeat clients who 'dip the stick' [of a pregnancy test] and call me," says Crystal Sada, a postpartum doula who serves clients in both New Jersey and Pennsylvania. "It is never too soon to plan. When a woman waits until the last month of her pregnancy to start making calls she usually finds her resources limited and sometimes no one is available for her. It also impacts the amount of time she has to get to know the doula and make a choice that is right for her and her family. When you start sooner, rather than later, you get to interview more doulas and find the right fit for you and your family."

# What Do You Want?

Knowing what you want before you begin your search is extremely important. Not every doula agrees about what a postpartum doula should or should not do. Some view their role as mentor and educator, but do not consider housework or cooking a part of the job description. Others offer more practical help, and of course, plenty fall somewhere in between.

To ensure a positive experience, think about what you want most from a postpartum doula, so you are able to ask the right questions on the phone or at an interview. Ask yourself the following questions:

- Why do you want to hire a postpartum doula?
- How many hours per day and how many days, weeks, or months do you plan on maintaining services?
- If perfection were possible, how would you define the perfect postpartum doula? How would you define an "acceptable" postpartum doula?

- Do you want a doula with personal mothering experience? Training? Certification? (Keep in mind that postpartum doula certification is relatively new, and there are many great doulas who are not certified.)
- Do you want a doula to help with housework? If yes, what type and how often?
- Do you want the doula to run errands?
- Do you want a doula to help with meal planning and cooking? Any special needs (for example, kosher, vegetarian, allergies)?
- Are there any religious considerations?
- Do you think you'll want overnight help with the baby, or do you expect to only have the doula during daylight hours?
- Do you expect the doula to help with older children? In what ways?
- Do you want the postpartum doula to help care for your pets?
- Are you expecting multiples?
- Do you anticipate any special problems, like postpartum depression? Recovery from cesarean birth? Special needs baby?
- Are you looking for a doula with any particular specialties (for example, infant massage, mother massage, kosher kitchen experience, counseling, preemies)?
- How much are you able to pay? Do you have any upper limits? (Fees range from $13 to $35 per hour.)

> "I wanted someone to do a lot of cooking, so I wanted to be upfront about that. I didn't anticipate needing a lot of education about baby care since I was already a registered nurse." —Jennifer, California

# Where to Look

Asking friends and family for referrals is always the first place to start. If you hired a labor doula, ask her. She may know people you can contact or agencies that you can call. You can ask your child-birth educator, local Le Leche League leaders, or your midwife or doctor. The labor and delivery department of a hospital or a nearby birth center may also have lists of postpartum doulas.

Most of the organizations that train or certify doulas provide referral services. Some have lists of local doulas on their Web sites, and others will mail you a list. Contact any of the following organizations, and ask them for a list of local postpartum doulas. (Be sure they know you want a *postpartum* doula, not a labor doula.)

Birth Works
P.O. Box 2045
Medford, NJ 08055
888-TO-BIRTH (862-4784)
email: info@birthworks.org
www.birthworks.org

CAPPA—Childbirth and Postpartum Professional Association
P.O. Box 491448
Lawrenceville, GA 30043
888-548-3672
email: info@cappa.net
www.cappa.net

CEF—Childbirth Enhancement Foundation
1004 George Ave.
Rockledge, FL 32955
321-631-9977
email: info@cefcares.org
www.cefcares.org

DONA—Doulas of North America
P.O. Box 626
Jasper, IN 47547
801-756-7331
email: doula@dona.org
www.dona.org

National Association of Postpartum Care Services
800 Detroit St.
Denver, CO 80206
800-45-DOULA
email: DoulaCare@aol.com
www.napcs.org

The Internet is another place to search. Type into any search engine the words "postpartum doula" and your state or city, and see what you find. You may actually discover the Web site of a local agency. Several Web sites offer searchable databases. Here are the best sites:

About.com's Pregnancy Resources
www.pregnancy.about.com/health/pregnancy/library/local/
    bllocalindex.htm

Birth Partners—Doulas
www.birthpartners.com

Doula Network
www.doulanetwork.com

DoulaWorld.com
www.doulaworld.com

The Labor of Love Pregnancy and Parenting Search Engine
www.thelaboroflove.com/websearch/links/Services/Doulas

Be sure to check the yellow pages of your local telephone directory, as some doulas advertise their services there.

There's a chance that there are no postpartum doulas in your area. If you find yourself in this situation, consider calling some local labor doulas, or childbirth educators, and asking if they are interested in doing some postpartum doula work. You may find someone who is interested in working for you, but would not necessarily advertise themselves as a postpartum doula to others.

# Interviewing

Depending on whether you go through a doula agency or hire privately, your interview experience will vary.

### HIRING FROM AN AGENCY

There are several advantages to hiring from a doula agency. The agency will be able to match you with someone quicker than if you looked for someone yourself, and the doulas will have been screened and received a certain level of training. Of course, this assumes that the agency is reputable!

Just as you would carefully interview a private doula, when hiring from an agency, you'll need to interview the owner or manger.

- *Check references.* The agency should be able to give you at least two different families to call as references. Ask if you can get references from the particular doula that the agency wants to assign to you.
- *Meet the doula before you sign or agree to services.* Not all postpartum doula agencies will assign the same doula for the entire service period, and some do not arrange an interview before services. You should always ask to meet before services begin. If this is not possible, request a phone interview.

- *Ask about training.* Are the doulas trained by the agency? Are they certified? By what organizations? What are the hiring requirements for this agency? Ask anything you would ask if you were hiring privately.
- *Ask about limitations and policies.* Some agencies do not allow doulas to drive their clients or client's families, for liability reasons. There are agencies that do not allow their doulas to do certain household tasks, like cleaning floors and bathrooms. Always ask about the agency's policies to make sure nothing conflicts with your needs and expectations.
- *Check with the Better Business Bureau (BBB).* You can search for the business at www.betterbusinessbureau.com. Keep in mind that the BBB only keeps businesses on file that either registered with the bureau or businesses for which a report was written. Not being listed at the Web site is neither a good nor bad sign.

If you decide to use a doula agency, you may be asked to fill out a form that asks key questions on your needs and preferences. From your answers, they then try to match you with an appropriate doula.

"When a person sends us what we call the 'Mother's Needs Outline,' describing what she anticipates her needs to be, and a $25 deposit to show she is serious and will not take our doulas' time just out of curiosity, we will match her up with a suitable doula to interview," explains Alice Gilgoff, owner and

"I interviewed only one other postpartum doula. The first doula I interviewed seemed inexperienced and had too much interest in my private life—mainly because she was so fascinated with pregnant women and birth."
—Laura, Oregon

founder of Mother Nurture, Inc., one of the first postpartum doula agencies in the United States. "This matchup may be based on who is available, or on geography (whether the doula is willing to travel to this client's community), but truly I try to match needs and abilities even more closely.

"For example, a doula who is a single mother may be asked to meet a client who will be a single mother herself. Or a doula who has had cesareans may interview with a client who has planned a repeat cesarean. The most unusual request I received was to find a doula with a compatible astrologic sign to the client's! I would say this is the main advantage in looking for a doula through an agency. That you have the opportunity to meet a doula for whom the matchup may show more of a thought process, whereas with a private doula, you will interview her, and if you wish to interview someone else, you'll have to go through the work of seeking new referrals from women in your community. We do not charge an additional $25 to have an interview with a second doula, if you've had a 'personality problem' with the first. By the way, I would say the overwhelming majority of clients choose the first doula they interview!"

## HIRING PRIVATELY

If you are looking for a postpartum doula who's working privately, not with the help of an agency, your first step is to call a few on the phone. (See appendix 3, an Interview Guide for Hiring a Postpartum Doula.) Be sure to ask about any special needs or requests you have. You'll want to ask questions like the following:

- Are you available the month of my due date? How many hours are you available per day? Per week?
- What kind of training and experience have you had?
- What is your personal parenting philosophy?
- What services do you provide? Do you provide night services?

- Are you willing to run errands? Drive the older children to school?
- What household chores do you usually help with?
- What do you charge for your services? How do you work out payment?
- Can you please give me the name and number of two previous clients, to call as references?
- Can we meet for a face-to-face interview? Do you charge a fee for this meeting?

Don't feel pressured to decide on the phone if you'd like to meet with this doula. Take your time, call others in the area, and check references or read over materials the doula may send you. "Ask the hard questions. Don't be afraid to talk about your fears or concerns with the doula," suggests Karen Schroeder, a postpartum doula from Michigan. "Also, ask reactive questions such as, what would you do if my child was choking? Listen to her answers, and then decide if you trust your child in the care of this doula."

Because your first meeting with a postpartum doula will occur in your home, you'll want to check her references before deciding to meet or hire her. It will only take ten minutes or less to call prior clients and ask about their experience. If your potential doula is not willing to

> "Pam told us, 'I basically take over the running of your household,' which were the words we had been waiting to hear. That, plus her demeanor and our hour-long interview, left us with no doubt." —Elizabeth, Oregon

give you even one person to call as a reference, take that as a red flag.

Unlike your first meeting with a labor doula, which is usually just an interview, a postpartum doula consultation meeting includes getting to know you, your family, your house, and sometimes includes

### ☙ A MOTHERING MOMENT . . .

"I was nervous about leaving the house and breastfeeding in public. Denise encouraged us to go for a walk to the local coffee house every day. Each day we'd go, get a drink, and sit in the café until the baby would begin to fuss. Denise would look at me and gently ask, 'Wanna try today?' I demurred several times. Then, one day, we decided to practice nursing the baby in her sling on my back porch, and it worked! I thought, 'Hey, I can do this!' Her gentle coaching gave me the confidence to try it out in public much sooner than I might have otherwise." —Jennifer, California

the doula giving advice and ideas on setting up the baby's room or other tips. You'll show her the laundry area and the kitchen. This will avoid her having to ask you questions after the baby is born and help her serve you better.

"After an initial contact, whether by phone or email, I will send out information: fees, references, estimated hours and 'what are your expectations of your doula' forms," says Marlene Gubler, a postpartum doula and Bradley childbirth teacher from Pennsylvania. "I will then do a free consultation visit in the last trimester of pregnancy for a tour of the home (washer/dryer, dishwasher, hampers) . . . I always offer references and encourage families to call. I encourage dads to talk with other dads to see how they can benefit as well."

As with a labor doula, the most important part of the interview is deciding if you feel comfortable with this person. "What you should look for is comfort," explains Gilgoff. "This is a person you have to feel free to 'hang out' with after the baby is born, and that may mean breasts hanging out, or asking her to launder your underwear that has a blood stain. Are you comfortable in front of this person? And

> "I think the most important issue is the personal fit. You are at a very emotionally poignant time in your life and want the person to add comfort, not make you feel like a stranger in your own home. I think the reason the person has chosen this line of work can give insight into whether they will fit your needs. My doula chose her work because she loves babies and loves being part of the special first days in a new family's life. She didn't depend on the income to support her family; rather it was a calling she felt."
> —Rachel, Missouri

do you feel her knowledge base is at the level you wish? Ask her key questions like 'How long should a baby breastfeed?' and see what she answers.

"Does she appear to be a person you can learn from, even if what you learn is, 'Do what you are comfortable with, what works for you as a family.' Ask her what she feels she can do for you, how she feels she will be a help to you. A doula should be your right-hand person, the person you can rely on to be your assistant, as if she were your best sister, or your ideal mom, available to meet your needs as they occur, and be respectful of your right to mother your baby in your own way."

"Women interviewing doulas should look for someone who will integrate herself into their home easily," explains postpartum doula Vicky York. "The doula she hires should be trained and certified, clean and healthy, mature and capable of the job. She should have experience with the issues the mom needs help with. She should share the mother's philosophy about parenting/living and support the mother's goals, agenda, and wishes—not just push her own. She should be available for the amount of time the mom needs or have a good backup. She should not have annoying habits like smoking or anything that would bother the particular mother. The mother should make sure the doula is willing to do the kind of housework she wants or needs. The doula should be friendly and accepting of the pets. She should be calm and reassuring, and most of all, both parents should like her."

# Contracts and Payment

Postpartum doulas are paid by the hour and the rates range from $13 up to $35. The rates will depend on where you live in the country and what services are being provided, with special nighttime care usually costing more than daytime services.

"Our doula was $20 an hour with a minimum four hours a week. We generally used about eight to twelve hours a week. We were very laid-back on tracking, billing, and payment. Generally, we squared up every other week, and sometimes bills were on a scrap of paper after we discussed what we thought the hours were. It worked for us, and we would not have changed it. But I could see where with someone else it would need to be more formal." —Shereen, Washington

"I charge $20 per hour, and yes, I do have sliding-scale and reduced fees," explains Crystal Sada, a postpartum doula working in Pennsylvania and New Jersey. "Some doulas charge more for multiples—actually I charge less. I am usually with these families for a longer period of time, and I know that I will be working several weeks and sometimes months with them. I try not to ever turn people away because they can't afford my fee. I am even willing to barter when I can, but at the same time, I need to make a living and pay my bills."

Some doulas ask that you commit to at least three hours of

"We signed an informal agreement that said we were responsible for payment, what the hourly rate was, and the minimum number of hours. Below the contract language was a checklist of chores and expectations—a type of roster of the things she might be doing. It was helpful. And even as informal as our arrangement was, I think a contract is a good idea." —Shereen, Washington

service for two days, or six hours of service, before they will add you as a client. Sometimes the fee for the first visit is paid before the baby is born in order to hold your spot and confirm to the doula that you are seriously interested in her services.

"I would be reluctant to advise a mom to sign a contract, unless the family is quite wealthy and can afford to use the doula whether they need her or not," says Kimberly Bepler, a doula in Oregon. "The needs of new families change by the day. I have found flexibility to be the name of the game."

However, a contract that does not commit you to a large number of hours is a good idea.

You'll want to have a contract that spells out the expectations of the doula's service and payment fees. It should address the following questions:

- What services will the doula provide?
- What services are not provided? (For example, if your doula will not chauffer members of your house around, it should be stated in the contract.)
- How many hours is your postpartum doula available? Is there a minimum amount of hours per day that she requires?

- What are the fees for each service? (For example: daytime service, $15 per hour, nighttime service, $20 per hour.)
- If you want nighttime care, what are the details of making that arrangement? (For example: how many hours, where will the doula sleep, how much will she be paid, and so on.)
- When should you call your doula to let her know you are ready for postpartum care, and how much notice is needed to arrange services?
- What amount are you required to pay in order for your doula to hold your due date on her calendar?
- How will the hours be tallied and how will payment be delivered?
- If the doula is not able to provide services because of illness or a family emergency, is there a backup? How will the payment schedule play out if the doula does call her backup?

There are a variety of different ways to arrange billing and payment schedules. "When I work for a family I am paid weekly—mostly by check," says Crystal Sada. "If the last day of the week I work is Friday, I get paid on Friday. If I work three days a week and the last day is Thursday then I expect to get paid on Thursday."

"I have a three-hour minimum, but for overnights it is an eight-hour minimum," explains Kimberly Bepler. "I bill at the end of the week, whatever the last day I worked was. I provide an invoice, with details of when I worked and how much I charged. I encourage couples to try to get reimbursement from insurance, which is why I provide them with this detailed invoice. Couples pay me mostly by checks, sometimes by cash. Occasionally I will bill for two weeks, but it is easier for them to remember what they are paying for if I bill weekly."

"I have two packages," says Gubler. "Package A is $16 per hour, strictly mother/baby care. It includes breastfeeding support; newborn care so mom can shower, rest, and eat; and sibling care. It doesn't include household chores except baby laundry. Package B, $18 per hour, includes all the above plus grocery stops, errands, family laundry (wash/fold/put away), kitchen tidy duties, meal prep, and family room tidying (no easy task with a few children/toddlers). I schedule my clients biweekly (two-week intervals) and bill my clients with an itemized receipt on the same biweekly schedule."

Postpartum doula care may seem expensive at first glance, but the help and faster healing is worth it. If you can only afford to have a postpartum doula for a couple of hours the first week after the birth, don't hesitate to call and ask what service packages they have available. If you can afford $150, that could add up to ten hours of service. You can spilt up those hours and have the doula come for two hours a day for five days. You can spread out beyond the five days if you think that will meet your needs best.

Speak with your family and decide what you can afford, and then figure out how many hours of service that would add up to and how often you'd like the help. You may be able to afford more hours than you realize, after you write everything down and do the math.

"The only thing that frustrates me more is when a mother wants or needs help after her baby is born and the family doesn't understand where she's coming from and thinks it's a waste of money," explains Gubler. "I find fathers to be a bit hesitant at times to hire doulas, but once they do, they are happy they did. I even had a doctor once tell a client of mine, 'What do you need a doula for? You don't need one of those; they are highly overrated.' Well, my client said to her doctor, 'Great, so then you will come to my home when my husband's at work and help with the two other children and newborn, so I can shower and nap?' After that, I don't think her doctor got on her case about having a doula again. In fact, I went with her to her six-week appointment, all the kids in tow, and he thought it was great. It was the first appointment he had with her without the kids playing in the room with all the equipment, and they were actually able to have a discussion uninterrupted."

# Third-Party Reimbursement

Receiving third-party reimbursement for postpartum doula services (such as from an insurance provider) may be easier than getting reimbursement for labor doula services, but you still may need to assert yourself to get the coverage. (See appendix 2 for a sample third-party reimbursement letter.) "I have had some reimbursement for my clients but it is far and few between," says Crystal Sada, a postpartum doula in Pennsylvania and New Jersey. "One mom had surgery two weeks after the birth of her fourth child and was not allowed to lift over ten pounds. Her baby weighted 10.4 at birth. Her surgeon and OB submitted letters, and it was paid for."

Here are some ways other moms received third-party reimbursement:

- *Send an invoice and insurance form to your insurance company, even if you know or think that they won't pay.* (See chapter 7 on hiring a labor doula for more information.) "I often encourage my clients to apply for insurance reimbursement," explains Kimberly Bepler, a postpartum doula. "I bill with a detailed invoice with the coverage codes printed on them, to allow my clients this option."
- Ask your doctor or midwife to write a letter explaining why you need a postpartum doula. Have them give a "prescription" for postpartum doula care. "The key is a good provider who understands what a doula is and does," Sada continues. "One OB wrote mom a letter for 'domestic help.' Well, that is just not going to get paid. Until our society understands the full ramifications of this work, I don't think insurance will pay anytime too soon."

  "Some [clients] have [had postpartum doula care covered by insurance], but they had very complicated deliveries and were referred by their OBs with paperwork to submit along with my bill," advises Rachel Silber, a certified childbirth educator, and labor and postpartum doula. "I encourage all women to try, only costs 37 cents to mail [the invoice] in, and the worst they can say is no!"

- If you give birth in a birth center, you may receive a certain number of postpartum doula services as a part of your labor and delivery package. If homebirth is covered by your insurance company, then postpartum doula services may also be paid for. Call the birth center, speak to your midwife, or call the insurance company and ask about postpartum doula coverage in these circumstances.

- If you plan on giving birth in a hospital, a postpartum doula may be paid for if you leave the hospital early, before 12 or 24 hours. Sometimes the hospital will offer a nurse for a one-time home visit, but not mention the option to use those funds towards a postpartum doula. Before you have the baby, call the hospital and ask about their early-discharge policies and procedures.

- Look into using your flexible spending accounts, if you or your partner has one, from your work place. "Many of my clients use flexible spending account reimbursements and all of them have been successful," says Silber.

- In *Mothering the New Mother* by Sally Placksin, the author relates that her husband's workplace paid for the doula. The husband told the company that he either wanted three weeks off of work, or they would have to pay for hired help during that time period to help his wife. The company paid for the doula so that the husband could continue working. Be sure to check with your own workplace; they may cover the doula care if it enables you to return to work sooner.

# PART FOUR

# The Antepartum Doula

## CHAPTER 12

# Introducing the Antepartum Doula

WHILE PREGNANCY IS A normal event for most women, every year more than 700,000 women are put on bed rest, for a variety of complications. Some are able to stay at home, while others must stay in a hospital. They are often on medications to prevent premature labor or to speed up the development of their child, in case premature birth does occur. This is a frightening time. A woman on bed rest is doing anything but resting. She is worried and nervous. She needs someone to talk to and someone to help explain the many options she has and procedures that may occur.

In a research study on bed rest, only 18 percent of the women felt that they were coping well emotionally and did not need outside help. About 50 percent of the women did not follow their doctor's bed rest order, either because they needed to take care of themselves or their families, or assumed that their condition was better. (Brown, 2002)

Until recently, a woman on bed rest was on her own, with no one in the birth professional world to help. But now, thanks to Diane Brown of the Childbirth and Postpartum Professional Association, antepartum doulas, or high-risk pregnancy labor supports, are available to provide informational, emotional, physical, and practical support to women during pregnancy.

"It's all about the baby, but what about mom? Someone to say you're doing great, what a wonderful job, what a good mother you are," explains Brown, founder and director of the antepartum doula program for CAPPA, and mother to three prematurely born children. "When on bed rest with my youngest son, I missed my second son's birthday. That was one of the most depressing moments in my life. I needed someone to say, 'Yes, but look what you are doing for your next child.' It all comes down to two words: empowerment and encouragement."

# Who Needs an Antepartum Doula?

"The antepartum client is different from the general pregnant population," says Laura Dana, a certified labor and antepartum doula in Florida. "She is faced with having to make decisions that can sometimes be life or death. She is typically more medically managed and because most parents are not experts in pregnancy, let alone a 'high-risk' one, she may or may not be fully informed enough to make decisions for her health and the health of her baby. What I do to help is to provide these moms with information regarding her particular situation, give her reading material, studies, or whatever is going to help her make sense of what is happening."

Women on bed rest are not the only ones who may benefit from antepartum doula support: Teen mothers, single women, rape victims, mothers with severe morning sickness, or any pregnant woman who finds herself in a difficult situation during pregnancy could receive guidance and practical help from an antepartum doula.

"Most of the mothers I work with are teens and really want and need someone supportive," says Michelle Cousins, an antepartum doula in Virginia. "Many clients like the companionship of someone who has been pregnant and need someone who knows what they are feeling. I also find that many mothers, especially first-time mothers, are embarrassed about certain aspects of pregnancy or just un-learned and feel embarrassed about asking certain questions. I never ridicule them for the questions they ask and always try to make them comfortable enough to share any and all feelings they have during their pregnancies.

"I worked with one teen who often called me about her boyfriend problems," continues Cousins. "She lived with her father and her mother was not in the picture. She saw me as a mother figure and often asked my opinions on things such as furniture choices, clothing, and even naming the baby. I was touched to have her think so highly of my thoughts and opinions."

# Antepartum Support

Antepartum doulas provide informational, emotional, physical, and practical support during pregnancy. They may also provide support during labor and the postpartum period, especially if a child is admitted to the neonatal intensive care unit.

If you are experiencing a high-risk pregnancy, you may feel overwhelmed, not knowing where to turn for help. Let's take a closer look at how an antepartum doula can help you.

### INFORMATIONAL SUPPORT

You may have many questions that even the more comprehensive pregnancy books do not answer completely. An antepartum doula is trained to help with high-risk pregnancies and will be able to either answer your questions, lend you books to read, or help you find the right professional to ask.

"I have an extensive lending library as well as access to many pamphlets and other information," says Cousins. "I always give a call-anytime card so they know they can talk to me when they need to. I will go with them to meetings and doctor appointments if they

**☙ A BIRTHING MOMENT . . .**

"I worked with a mom whose amniotic sac ruptured at 26 weeks. She was a healthy woman, second pregnancy, but obviously if she had delivered at 26 weeks her baby would have faced many challenges. She was sequestered in the hospital in the high-risk unit to try to eek out as much time as possible. She was very well educated about her health, but unfamiliar about her choices and what she could expect. I provided her with books to read regarding premature labor and birth as well as research and statistical information about the time element in regard to her ruptured membranes. I made frequent visits while she sat in the hospital away from her family (a husband and a 6-year-old son who lived too far away to visit daily) and checked in on her by phone every few days. Fortunately, she was a very compliant patient, hungry for information, and maintained her pregnancy until 34 weeks when an induction was scheduled. She delivered a small but healthy baby boy after many hours of Pitocin and never used any pain medications throughout the 19-hour induction. Even though he had to remain in the hospital for a little while, this mom was empowered to do what she needed for herself in the labor and for him after the birth, including breastfeeding." —Laura Dana, Florida

desire and help them write a birth plan if they desire. I sometimes talk with other members of the family and help them through the adjustments they are making or may need to make."

You may not be able to attend childbirth education classes if you're on bed rest. An antepartum doula can teach you and your partner a private childbirth education course. An antepartum doula can also provide all the support a labor doula provides, if you choose to hire her for your birth as well. An antepartum doula will be more familiar with the protocols and procedures used in high-risk birth.

## EMOTIONAL SUPPORT

Emotional support may be the most important part of antepartum doula support. When you're on bed rest, it's difficult to think of anything besides your unborn child and the neverending list of what-ifs. Also, not being able to do things for yourself or your family can be frustrating and upsetting. Your antepartum doula can talk to you about your concerns and worries, and she will provide you with the encouragement that you need.

"I place a great deal of emphasis on a woman's inner knowing, ask a lot of questions, and help to seek answers with her," explains Jesse Remer Henderson of Mother Tree Doula Services in Oregon. "I use education as a catalyst rather than a definitive 'right answer' so that a woman comes to conclusions herself. Information is much

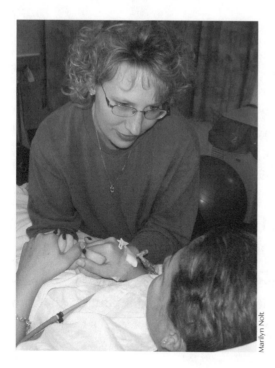

FIGURE 12.1. Hand in hand, a mother receives moral support from her doula.

Marilyn Nolt

more powerful when based in insight and breakthroughs. And pregnancy opens women both physically and hormonally to that space within their own power."

Talking over your concerns is just one way your doula can help. Feeling pampered can really lift your spirits. Some doulas will do your hair or bring you rented videos and pop some popcorn.

"I provide a lot of comfort measures," explains Henderson, "listening, massage, aromatherapy, teas. These are catalysts for self-growth for a woman as she learns about her changing body and how to prepare for the unexpected yet certain outcome of her birth."

### PHYSICAL SUPPORT

Antepartum doulas can teach you relaxation, which is important for labor, as well as for emotional well-being anytime. Your doula may be able to give you a hand or foot massage. Helping you with your practical needs will encourage you to stay off your feet when it is necessary.

### PRACTICAL SUPPORT

An antepartum doula provides the same type of practical support that a postpartum doula provides. She may cook meals, organize, tidy the house, do laundry, wash dishes, and run errands. If you're in the hospital, your doula may be able to help around your home and then come to see and speak with you. Read chapter 10 for more on how doulas help with practical needs.

# How to Hire an Antepartum Doula

Antepartum doulas have not been around long, and very few certified and trained antepartum doulas are available. But postpartum and labor doulas were providing antepartum services even before certification and training programs existed. Even if there are no certified antepartum doulas in your area, there may be other birth professionals willing to serve you.

The first place to look is on the Childbirth and Postpartum Professional Association (CAPPA) Web site at www.cappa.net. Or you can call 888-548-3672. CAPPA is the first and only national doula organization to recognize and train antepartum doulas. They will be the best people to contact first in your search.

If you have no success with CAPPA, then start calling childbirth educators, your doctor's office, the antepartum unit at the hospital, and local postpartum and labor doulas. Ask around, and see if anyone has experience with this work. You can also try searching one of the following Web sites:

About.com's Pregnancy Resources
www.pregnancy.about.com/health/pregnancy/library/local/
    bllocalindex.htm

Birth Partners—Doulas
www.birthpartners.com

Doula Network
www.doulanetwork.com

DoulaWorld.com
www.doulaworld.com

The Labor of Love Pregnancy and Parenting Search Engine
www.thelaboroflove.com/websearch/links/Services/Doulas

Just like interviewing for a postpartum or labor doula, call people, ask questions, and decide if you'd like to meet with them. You can find an antepartum doula interview guide in appendix 4 of this book. Questions you may consider asking include:

- What kind of doula training and experience have you had?
- How many hours are you available per day? Per week?
- Do you have any personal experience with [your problem here]?
- What services do you provide? Do you provide labor or post-partum doula services?
- Are you willing to run errands? Drive older children to school? What household chores do you usually help with?
- What do you charge for your services? How do you work out payment?
- Can you please give me the name and number of two previous clients, to call as references?
- Can we meet for a face-to-face interview? Do you charge a fee for this meeting?

"Personally, I would be more interested in finding someone who had 'been there, done that,' so to speak," says doula Laura Dana. "A doula who has had personal experience with bed rest, hospitalization, tocolytic medications, high-risk concerns, and so on would probably be better equipped to help another woman in the same situation. I would ask about a lending library, if the doula had the ability to teach childbirth education since most likely a high-risk mom is not going to be able to make classes, and what services she provided in the antepartum period. I would also ask if she was equipped to follow the pregnant mom through to labor and birth."

Antepartum doulas are usually paid by the hour, around the same fee range as postpartum doulas: $15 to $30 per hour. "I do have a contract that I sit down and discuss with the client mom/couple," explains doula Laura Dana. "It spells out my role, my responsibilities, my limitations, and it also does the same for the client. Payment is handled on an individual basis. I never want my clients to have to make a decision between paying the electric bill and paying me, so I will work out whatever payment arrangement they need. I let them know that this is how I make my living, but I am able to make it work for them.

"I assisted a mom who was an insulin dependant gestational diabetic," continues Dana. "She and her husband thought that hiring a doula was very important since this was her second go-around with gestational diabetes and she wanted to remain as 'normal' as possible going into her labor and birth. They didn't have a lot of money to spare, but we worked out a $50 a week payment plan. This was what worked for them, and fortunately for me, they really stuck to it."

"I usually take a deposit of the first week's pay after a schedule has been established and an agreement signed by the family," explains doula Jesse Henderson. "On the contract, I include details of what we've discussed so that we are both clear on expectations. If the antepartum is inclusive of birth, I include two of those visits as part of a birth package along with two postpartum visits and then follow up with hourly rates for additional time."

If you do not end up finding an antepartum doula, your search was not in vain. Just by calling local doulas and other birth professionals and asking for antepartum doula services, you are encouraging more people to go into this much-needed birth support profession. As more people request antepartum services, more doulas will become certified and trained to provide support.

PART FIVE

# Becoming a Doula

CHAPTER 13

# Becoming
# a Doula

So you want to become a doula. Perhaps you had a wonderful experience with your doula, and now you want to help other women have positive birth or postpartum experiences. Or maybe you have never had children, but love working with new mothers and their babies. Whatever your reason, you are joining a special and diverse group, who all share at least one goal: to support women and their families during pregnancy, childbirth, and the postpartum period.

All kinds of people become doulas: young mothers, grandmothers, single mothers, childless women. Some women become a doula because they eventually want to work as a labor and delivery nurse or as a midwife. Alternatively, some nurses and midwives work as doulas later in their career.

"I have had amazing women attend my workshops, from new nursing students who are just learning about birth to incredibly experienced doulas who feel the need for formal certification," says Connie Banack, who trains childbirth educators, labor doulas, and postpartum doulas for the Childbirth and Postpartum Professional Association (CAPPA). "I have learned from every woman who has attended my workshops, especially those who have had or are planning

## ❧ DOULA REFLECTIONS . . .

"I became an antepartum doula because of my own experience of being a high-risk pregnant mom. I had two twin pregnancies, 18 months apart, the first of which ended tragically when our fraternal twin daughters were born and died at 25 weeks. During the following months when my husband and I resumed our quest to become pregnant, I began reading everything that I could get my hands on in regard to pregnancy. I was obsessed with gaining as much information as possible. I began peer counseling for a grief support group called CLIMB (Center for Loss In Multiple Birth) and through that organization, I was able to help other parents who had experienced multiple birth loss at all gestational periods. I provided parents with information, support, and practical advice about getting through the grieving period—very much what a doula does in pregnancy. Once my husband and I became pregnant again, this time with fraternal twin boys, we knew that my pregnancy would be very high-risk considering my history. At 17 weeks, I required a cerclage to hold my cervix shut, complete bed rest, and by 26 weeks, I was admitted to the antepartum unit at one of the local hospitals. It was a nighttime nurse who acted as my doula. She held my hand when I was scared, she talked to me to keep me distracted, and she provided me with information to help me make better-informed choices." —Laura Dana, Florida

a VBAC (vaginal birth after cesarean), as they often are very motivated to support women in avoiding unnecessary cesareans or towards successful VBACs."

"Many women come into the trainings thinking that they will go on to midwifery," explains Ilana Stein, a certified birth doula trainer.

"By the time they finish, they often realize that doula work is exactly what they want to be doing and then do not pursue further training. They find enormous satisfaction in the work."

Now is one of the best times to become a doula. There are a variety of organizations who offer training and certification, and even if you are unable to attend a training, there are now distance learning programs and videos available. Plus there is a great need for antepartum, labor, and postpartum doulas. While you can usually find at least one or two labor doulas within an hour's driving distance, more locally based postpartum and antepartum doulas are in great need.

# Should You Become a Doula?

Do you have what it takes? As wonderful and fulfilling as doula work can be, the profession can also be draining, difficult, and expensive. Before you decide to become a doula, consider your current family needs, if you are financially capable, if your day job is flexible, and if you are physically and emotionally healthy.

### YOUR FAMILY'S NEEDS

If you have young children, you'll need to carefully consider if doula work is right for you at this time in your life. If you plan on working as a labor doula, you may be away for long periods of time and need to leave in the middle of the night. If you're breastfeeding your baby or co-sleeping, consider how your child will react if you're away for a long period of time. I'm not saying it's impossible to work as a labor doula under these circumstances, but you'll certainly need reliable last-minute babysitting and a supportive family.

If you're bent on becoming a doula, but are a mother of young children, you may want to consider postpartum or antepartum doula work. You'll have more control over what hours you work, and you can work as few or as many hours as you decide to commit to your clients.

"I originally wanted to be a labor doula, but didn't feel that I could be gone a long time from my children, because I was still breastfeeding," says Wendy Middleton, a certified postpartum doula, labor doula, lactation educator, and postnatal educator. "So I decided to try working for a short time as a postpartum doula and loved it! Eventually I became a labor doula and antepartum doula as well. Five years later, I am still doing postpartum support, and love the flexibility and great rewards this career offers."

Also consider how supportive your partner will be. Especially with labor doula work, you may be receiving calls in the middle of the night, feel exhausted after long births, or feel drained after working with moms in difficult situations. If your partner does not support your work, you are bound to have relationship problems as time goes on.

## SALARY EXPECTATIONS

Doulas are generally underpaid. If insurance companies would pay for services and recognize the worth of doulas, then perhaps this work would be a profitable profession. However, in order to allow families to afford doulas, the cost of services remains relatively low compared to the amount of hours, training, and various expenses. Very few doulas are able to make a real living out of this work, and you'll be one of few if you make more than $15,000 a year. Many doulas just break even or even go into debt, if they are not serious about the business aspects of doula work.

"As she is trying to start up a doula service, I would remind her that like any business, she will need to spend money to make money," explains Middleton. Startup expenses include books to study, training seminars, childbirth education, lactation and newborn baby care classes, membership dues to a doula organization, and certification and application fees. Add in a cell phone and pager service, advertisement costs, various business paraphernalia, like business cards

> ## 🐾 DOULA REFLECTIONS . . .
>
> "I was looking to do some work part-time as my third child was approaching her fourth birthday, knowing she would be going to school full-time in a matter of a few short years. Literally the day after she turned four, I saw an article in the *New York Times* about a group of women running a postpartum doula agency in Manhattan. Although the work was very different from what I was thinking of doing, it spoke to me. I loved being around babies, and I knew I wouldn't be having any more of my own. I carefully researched the idea of being a doula, attended a DONA conference in Cleveland, read a lot of books, and about 18 months later opened the doors to Mother to Mother. It is now five years later. I worked the first four years by myself and a little over a year ago trained five women to work with me." —Barbara J. Coscia, Connecticut

and information packets, birth and comfort supplies, and legal costs of registering your business name with the government.

It is possible to make over $20,000 a year, but it will take a great deal of organization, business smarts, and determination. "I think it takes a few things [to make over $20,000]," explains Teresa Howard, a certified labor doula, lactation educator, and childbirth educator who makes over $20,000 a year in profits. "Volume is one thing: you must do four births a month at $500 each in order to make $24,000 in revenue as a doula. I think it helps to be incorporated so you have some tax advantages. I also think it helps to sell some products. I sell slings, baby shoes, and birth balls as well as breastfeeding products like bras, sore nipple products, and breastfeeding pillows. I also teach childbirth classes. I think you can do it just doing births as a labor doula, but you must either charge a lot more than $500 or do additional things that compliment being a doula."

## FLEXIBILITY

Some doulas are stay-at-home mothers or retired women who decided to try this. On the other hand, plenty of women who want to be doulas need to work to supplement their family's income (or to support their doula work!).

If you plan on working as a postpartum or antepartum doula, having an additional job besides your doula work should not be too difficult, though your boss will need to be open to you receiving phone calls during work hours. Obviously, you'd need to decide how many hours you can serve as a doula without feeling overwhelmed or overworked, so that you can give your clients the attention and enthusiasm that they deserve.

If you plan on working as a labor doula, you'll need a job that will allow you to leave at a moment's notice, and perhaps, a job that will allow you to be out of the office for a day or so after long or difficult births. (So you won't worry that your client is taking "too long" to give birth, and so you can get your rest.)

Some doulas work in groups and assign on call-hours. If you can arrange this with other local doulas, then you can schedule your work around your on-call hours. However, doulas rarely start off working in a formal group, and you may need to get through training and at least your first year on your own. If you plan on volunteering at a hospital or birth center, they may also have on-call hours for doulas, and they are usually more willing to train and hire new doulas.

## PHYSICAL AND EMOTIONAL HEALTH

Doula work requires good health. As a labor doula, you'll need to be able to stay awake for as long as your client needs you, to get up at 3 A.M., and perhaps not get back home to your bed until 20 hours later. While you should be sure to bring snacks and drink plenty of water during a birth, you may not have a real meal for hours at a time. Some births are easy, but some are long and difficult, and you need to be able to handle both.

You'll need to be able to provide massage or deep and constant counterpressure to the back, help hold a woman in a squat position, or allow her to rest her weight on you while she stands during contractions. You could work with another doula, but most mothers prefer as few people as possible supporting her during birth. Of course, you should never work without a backup doula who you can call to replace you for a break when a birth is long or difficult. But you should be able to support a mother for at least 16 hours (the average time for a first birth) without needing to call a backup.

"Once, I was called in to a birth in the middle of the afternoon, and supported the family for 13 hours of labor," tells Middleton. "In the wee hours of the morning, just as I was finishing up, I received a page. It was another client in labor who was just getting to the same hospital. I went two doors down and helped this family through a 30-hour labor! It was a tough labor and required a lot of strenuous physical work from me. When I was approaching 40 hours without sleep, I began to get a little delirious! So I called my backup doula, and she relieved me while I took a catnap in another room, to restore myself for supporting the family through transition and pushing. It was a 43-hour shift I'll never forget!"

You won't be able to work with a newborn if you're always getting sick. And you must be physically strong. New mothers sometimes need help getting in and out of bed after difficult births, as do high-risk moms on bed rest. Both postpartum and antepartum doulas are on their feet doing as much as they can for the new or bedridden expectant mother, in usually a short period of time. Never underestimate the amount of stress on your back and muscles from picking up, rocking, or carrying a newborn baby or toddler.

Emotional health is just as important. Your priority when serving women during pregnancy, childbirth, and/or the postpartum

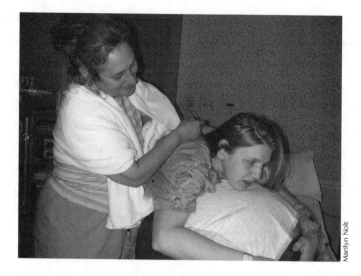

Marilyn Nolt

FIGURE 13.2 With a smile on her face,
this doula takes pleasure in her work.

period should be to support and empower them and aid them in achieving their goals. If you become a doula in order to push what you consider to be the "perfect birth" experience, or the parenting style that you think is best, or any other type of personal agenda, then you are doing a disservice to your clients.

Consider whether you are going into doula work to deal with your own loss or negative birth or mothering experiences. Don't get me wrong: Many great doulas originally went into the profession as a result of personal negative experiences. But it's important to keep in mind the needs of your clients and not impose on them what you wish your experience had been. For example, if you ended up with a medicated birth, when you wanted a birth without interventions, you may find yourself pushing women to have nonmedicated births, even when that is not what's best for them in their situation, or what they desire for their birth experience. Becoming aware of your motives, and learning how to support clients who may not share your birth or parenting philosophies, is the first step to becoming a great doula.

I don't want to discourage anyone. But it's important to understand the potential challenges. If after consideration, you think you are capable and ready to work as a doula, then it's time to start your lifelong education and training.

# Six Traits That All Great Doulas Must Have

1. **Self-motivation.** Unless you join a hospital or volunteer doula training program, no one is going to be there to make sure you read the books that are required, attend the classes and training, and keep your doula business going. An internal drive is extremely important.

2. **A desire for lifelong learning.** Doulas never stop learning. After you complete the initial training and recommended reading lists, you should continue to read books, attend conferences, and constantly take advanced doula classes. You must also be open to learning from every client and every doula that you meet, and avoid thinking that you have nothing more to learn. Some doulas look at other doulas as competition instead of co-workers, and this attitude prevents them from learning as much as they can.

3. **Perceptiveness.** A woman will not always be able to articulate her needs. You'll need to be perceptive and anticipate her needs. "This professional field is so new that sometimes we have to teach our clients how to use our services," says Vicky York, a postpartum doula trainer. "A postpartum doula should be able to see what seems to need to be done, make suggestions, and do the logical thing."

4. **Passion.** "When I train women to be doulas," explains Kathy Clark, a certified doula trainer in Colorado, "I have the opportunity to interact with them very closely, and I feel I can usually identify those women who have what I call the

doula heart. It's a passion I can see when they are learning techniques, asking questions, practicing techniques on one another. They are like sponges, and the more they do and learn, the more they just glow! The ones who stand back and watch and don't interact are generally (in my experience) the ones who are looking for a way to make money. They don't have the passion."

5. **Flexibility.** Your job is to help your client feel positive and empowered, even if the birth does not go as planned. You won't be able to do this if you remain set either on your client's birth plan, or if you push your personal agenda.

"Many doulas lose sight of the bigger picture," says Debbie Lavin, certified labor doula and trainer. "When I attend doula meetings, many times I hear these two comments: 'I haven't had a medicated birth in x-many months (or years).' This statement clearly indicates that the success of these births belongs to the doula when it should belong to the mom. It also reveals that the doulas who make these statements may have been asserting their own agenda and failing to see their role in supporting a woman and her choices. The other commonly stated comment I hear is, 'The mom needed pain meds so I feel like a failure.' Again, this reveals that the doula is taking responsibility for the outcome. The risk in this viewpoint is that the doula has lost sight of the bigger picture and probably missed many opportunities to point out all the other successful and powerful aspects of that particular birth, and most especially, of the mother and her partner. The best part of being a doula is that there are always opportunities for empowerment to be revealed as long as the doula has this as her goal, rather than just keeping a mom from using pain medications."

"Birth and this profession are very unpredictable," says Kathryn Berkowitz, a certified labor and postpartum doula

**DOULA REFLECTIONS . . .**

"I used to work as a union organizer, which is a very demanding job! After my son was born in '98 I went back to work for nine months and it was very difficult, so I changed careers entirely. I set out to get certified as a childbirth educator with the Bradley Method, a doula through DONA, and a breastfeeding counselor. This way, I could stay home with my son full-time and still do work that was meaningful to me. I really find it useful to be a doula in addition to a childbirth educator because you have the firsthand experience as a labor assistant to share ideas and stories with your students. Doing doula work has led me to consider a midwifery career but I've decided against it because I have come to realize that what I love about birth is more about supporting the women as they become mothers, and supporting the partners as they become parents as well. I like being able to focus on that entirely at a birth; the midwife has many more responsibilities in addition to supporting the mom." —Jane Cruice, Pennsylvania

trainer. "A doula must be willing to give up family holidays. . . . Being on call 24-7 for four weeks at a time for each client is not something one can fully appreciate unless they have done it. A smart doula will anticipate her calendar and book clients accordingly, and know when to refer and work cooperatively with other doulas in her area for backup, etc."

6. **Professionalism.** Being professional means taking your education and business practices seriously. It means attending clients on time, dressing appropriately, listening to their thoughts, and supporting their needs, even if it goes against

your personal philosophy. It means not gossiping about fellow doulas, nurses, or care providers, and it means respecting your client's right to confidentiality. Always remember that when you attend a client, their families, friends, and care providers will judge all other doulas by your example.

"Being a doula is an honor," says Clark. "Almost anyone can find an opportunity to be at a birth but when you participate as a doula, regardless of the specifics, you have been invited to witness the birth of a family. It is a sacred time, one that cannot be replaced or redone, no matter how many children this mother has. It is your responsibility to be the eyes, ears, and hands that are the 'gatekeepers' of this momentous occasion. You see the mom's first look at her child; you hear the first words spoken; see the way the baby looked, moved, etc.; and your hands will help encourage this mother through her pain, her work, and even putting her baby against her skin. This is a responsibility you should take seriously. Document it and give it to the family as a helpful remembrance of the moments of birth that they may not have been able to notice."

# Training

There are a variety of paths to become a doula. Some doulas start their training with no formal education or personal experience in motherhood or pregnancy, while others are veteran childbirth educators or seasoned grandmothers. National organizations provide training and certification programs, with many offering different programs depending on your previous education and experience.

Certification from a national doula organization usually involves becoming a member of the organization and then completing a list of requirements, which always includes attending a doula training or watching a video of a live seminar. Some organizations require you to take an exam (usually open-book) or write a book or topic report. You may also need to attend a certain amount of births, or work a certain number of hours, and then have your client and other members of the birth team or family fill out an evaluation.

Visit Web sites of doula organizations to review what is required for certification and find out if there is training in your area, or if a distance learning program is offered. Compare the various organizations. They have different philosophies, different costs, and different benefits.

ALACE—Association of Labor Assistants and Childbirth
    Educators
P.O. Box 382724
Cambridge, MA 02238
617- 441-2500
email: alacehq@aol.com
www.alace.org

BBI—Birth and Bonding International
1126 Solano Ave.
Albany, CA 94706
510-527-2121
email: bbint@flash.net
www.birthbonding.org

Birthing from Within
123 Wellesley SE
Albuquerque, NM 87106
505-254-4884
email: contact@birthingfromwithin.com
www.birthpower.com

Birth Works
P.O. Box 2045
Medford, NJ 08055
888-TO-BIRTH (862-4784)
email: info@birthworks.org
www.birthworks.org

CAPPA—Childbirth and Postpartum Professional Association
P.O. Box 491448
Lawrenceville, GA 30043
888-548-3672
email: info@cappa.net
www.cappa.net

CEF—Childbirth Enhancement Foundation
1004 George Ave.
Rockledge, FL 32955
321-631-9977
email: info@cefcares.org
www.cefcares.org

DONA—Doulas of North America
P.O. Box 626
Jasper, IN 47547
801-756-7331
email: doula@dona.org
www.dona.org

ICEA—The International Childbirth Education Association
P.O. Box 20048
Minneapolis, MN 55240
952-854-8660 or 800-827-ICEA
email: info@icea.org
www.icea.org

National Association of Postpartum Care Services
800 Detroit St.
Denver, CO 80206
800-45-DOULA
email: DoulaCare@aol.com
www.napcs.org

There are many advantages of certifying with a doula organization: You will receive referrals, get discounts on continuing education credits and conferences, and be recognized as a professional. But certification is not always necessary or possible. Certainly, many great doulas have never received certification. Doulas have existed long before national organizations set up certification programs! Some doulas do not want to sign an organization's position or scope of practice declarations, something all certifying organizations require. Plus, the cost of certification can be prohibitive, with membership and application fees costing hundreds of dollars.

"Though certification shows that a doula has the basic knowledge needed to support women in childbirth, many incredibly knowledgeable doulas choose not to certify for many reasons," explains Connie Banack, a certified doula, childbirth educator, and doula trainer. "Only a client should have the right to decide if a doula is qualified for them and that has to be respected by every birth professional."

If you decide not to attain certification, for whatever reason, you'll need to be diligent that you receive the same, and perhaps even more, education than those that choose certification. You can attend a doula training or watch a doula training video without completing a certification program. You should meet the requirements for certification, even if you don't send in membership dues or formally apply.

"I'd suggest looking to the requirements of a program as a model," says Wendy Middleton, a certified postpartum doula trainer and lactation educator trainer with CAPPA. "They should do lots of reading, watch videos, research topics such as breastfeeding challenges and postpartum depression, and ask their clients to fill out evaluations, so they can get feedback. I would also recommend that they inform themselves on all local resources for the childbearing family and become members of such organizations as La Leche League, Postpartum Support International, and the Childbirth and Postpartum Professionals Association."

Whether you intend to receive certification or not, here are ways you can become one of the best educated doulas in your city:

- *Read.* Read everything you can find about pregnancy, birth, postpartum recovery, breastfeeding, and motherhood. Read the books that are required for other certification programs, even if you do not need to read that particular book for your program. Read books that you disagree with, so you know what your potential clients are reading. You don't need to spend a lot of money to read books. You can visit used-book stores and public libraries. Birth centers and hospitals also provide lending libraries.

  "Read everything you can about birth, learn from everyone—from Michel Odent to Penny Simkin," says Banack. "Learn their philosophies of birth and apply their years of wisdom to your practice as you support birthing families. Certification is only the beginning of an amazing journey toward empowering women in this generation and creating better birth experiences for them and their babies."

- *Network.* Find local doulas, and find out if there is a local network of birth educators. If there does not yet exist a doula group for your city or state, consider starting one. Go to meetings, talk to people, and find out who is in your community. This is a good way to meet other doulas who may work as your partners in the future, and also a great way to exchange ideas and get inspired by others in the birth field.

DOULA REFLECTIONS . . .

"The inspiration to become a doula started with a simple interest in the stories told to me by a friend who is an OB nurse. I became more and more interested in being a part of the whole labor and delivery process. I then discovered that my own cousin had recently become a certified doula. I hired my cousin to help me at the birth of my son, and three weeks after giving birth, I attended my doula training. One year later I received my certification through DONA, and now I have my doula business and also do volunteer doula care at a local hospital." —Kimberly Govekar, Oregon

Often, doula groups are able to bring in speakers, something you cannot do on your own or without a network in place.

- *Attend conferences and continuing education programs.* Almost every doula organization sponsors a conference once a year. Usually you need to pay for the conference, but CAPPA's conferences are free to members. Even if you have to travel and it's difficult for you, consider going at least every other year, if you can't go once a year. Be sure to also sign up for advanced training classes that may be offered by doula organizations.
- *Observe local childbirth education and newborn education classes.* Attend local support groups, like La Leche League or postpartum depression support groups, at least once, so you can see what you can recommend to your clients. Try to observe more than one type of childbirth method. For example, if you're familiar with the Bradley method, sit in on a hospital-based Lamaze class or a Birthing from Within class. Know what your clients are learning, pick up new tips and

tricks, and observe the classes with an open mind and an open notebook.

- *Learn from everyone.* Never consider yourself an expert, because as soon as you do, you'll find yourself ignoring other people's good advice and wisdom. Learn from your clients and learn from other doulas.

- *Find a doula to mentor you.* Call your doula trainer or look up local doulas and ask if they or anyone in the area might be willing to act as your mentor. You can start off by attending births with them (with the permission of their clients of course). Slowly, your mentor should be able to help you become more involved. There is no better way to learn how to act as a doula than by watching and aiding an experienced doula.

- *Join online email lists or message boards for doulas.* You can ask many questions about starting your journey, and ask about the various paths to doula-ship. One of the most helpful lists I have found online is the Fen's Ende doula list: www.fensende.com/Users/swnymph/email.html. There are message boards for doulas at ParentsPlace.com and MotheringMagazine.com. You also can search www.groups .yahoo.com for doula support groups.

## LIFELONG LEARNING

Your journey to become a doula does not end after you receive your certification papers or after you finish an apprenticeship with another doula. The good doulas are constantly learning, always trying to help their clients feel more confident, informed, and empowered. Every day, more research is carried out, and more books are written. You must seek out all of this information, even if you don't agree with the findings or opinions. Most importantly, learn from every woman you support, every birth you attend, every family that you serve.

Take this book and read the sections on doula support over and over, to see the many ways you can offer support to women. Talk to mothers in your family, and those you meet in the malls or at the park, and ask them: What did they need most during birth? What did they need most after their babies were born? Use the information you gather from fellow doulas, other birth and breastfeeding professionals, and the women you support to become the best doula you can be. Whether you act as a doula for ten or fifty women a year, remember that you will make difference in the world, one family at a time.

# Appendix 1
## Interview Guide for Hiring a Labor Doula

F<small>EEL FREE TO PHOTOCOPY</small> this questionnaire to help interview potential doulas. The questions are only a guideline. You may have questions not listed below, or some questions here may not be relevant to your situation. For more detailed information on hiring a labor doula, see chapter 7.

## Phone Interview Guide

Name of Doula: _____

Phone number (_____)_____-_____

E-mail address: _____

Additional contact information: _____

_____

If the doula says this is a bad time, schedule to call another time.

Date: _____ Time: _____

QUESTIONS TO ASK DURING PHONE INTERVIEW:

1. What kind of training and experience as a doula have you had?

_____

_____

_____

2. What is your personal childbirth philosophy?

_____

_____

_____

3. Please tell me about the services you offer?

_____

_____

_____

4. What do you charge for your services? Do you offer payment
   plans?

_____

_____

_____

5. Are you willing to meet with me at home before I go to the
   hospital/birth center? OR Do you have experience with home-
   births, and are you willing to attend one?

_____

_____

_____

6. Can you provide me with a couple names and phone numbers of
   previous clients, for references?

_____

_____

_____

ADDITIONAL QUESTIONS AND NOTES:

_____

_____

_____

_____

If you decide to meet with the doula in-person:
When: _____

Where you plan to meet with your doula: _____

Directions to the meeting place: _____

_____

# Doula Interview Guide

Use this as a guide when you meet with any potential doulas. While part of your goal is to find out what services this doula offers, the most important part of the interview is to decide if her personality is a good fit. Do you feel comfortable with her? Do you like her?

Name of Doula: _____

Phone number (_____)_____-_____

E-mail address: _____

Additional contact information: _____

_____

When asking these questions, pay more attention to her way of speaking, her personality and her overall attitude, than to her specific answers.

- Why did you go into doula work?
- (If she is a mother herself) Can you tell me about the most difficult part of the birth of your child(ren)? What birth memory do you cherish most?
- What is the most challenging aspect of your work as a doula?
- What do you see as your main role at my birth?
- How will you help my partner/family at the birth?
- I'm planning a medicated birth/homebirth/non-medicated birth. Do you have experience supporting clients who choose this option? Can you tell me how you typically support these clients?

## DETAILS OF HER SERVICES:

Do you include any prenatal visits? How many, and what do you usually do with your clients at the prenatal meetings?

_____

_____

_____

At what point do you join me in my labor? How do I contact you? Can I expect you to be available during the two weeks before and after my expected due date?

_____

_____

_____

Do you have a back-up doula? If yes, under what circumstances do you call her? Can I meet with her before the birth? Can I have her contact information?

_____

_____

_____

Do you offer any optional or extra services? (Photography, video, belly casting, etc.) How much do these extra services cost, or are they included in the overall price?

_____

_____

_____

What comfort measures do you typically use at a birth? And what do you usually bring to a birth, to help your clients? (For example, a birth ball, massage oils, etc.)

_____

_____

_____

How long after the birth will you be available? Do you help with breastfeeding? What type of support do you provide postpartum?

_____

_____

_____

What are the terms of your contract? What do I need to pay to hold my date? What are the payment terms?

_____

_____

_____


## NOTES FOR ANY SPECIAL QUESTIONS YOU HAVE:
*(Tip: Write down any special questions here before you go to the meeting.)*

_____

_____

_____

_____

_____

_____

_____

_____

# Appendix 2
## Third-Party Reimbursement Letter

Even if you think your insurance company will not cover your doula expenses, apply anyway. If more women apply for reimbursement, insurance companies may consider adding the service to their coverage list.

First, ask your doula to send an invoice to your insurance company. You can find an invoice at www.dona.org/PDF/3PRDoulaInvoice.pdf. Or you can call your insurance company and ask them to send you an application or invoice form.

Chances are, your claim will be denied. After you receive your denial, send a letter like the following to your insurance company. Obviously, the below is only a sample, and you will want to change it to fit your situation. Ask your doula to write a letter as well, and send your letter and your doula's letter together to your insurance company, along with whatever paperwork your insurance company requires for an appeal. Also consider sending a position paper, of either DONA or CAPPA, that outlines the research on doulas.

Position papers from CAPPA:
http://www.cappa.net/CAPPA_Position_Paper_CBE.asp

Position papers from DONA:
http://www.dona.org/PDF/BDPositionPaper.pdf
http://www.dona.org/PDF/PDPositionPaper.pdf

SAMPLE LETTER:
[Your name and return address here]
[Date here]

[Company name and address here]

To Whom It May Concern:

I hired a doula to support me during my pregnancy. Several research studies have shown that doulas contribute to less interventions and more positive birth experiences. Labor doulas help women avoid c-sections and have faster births, which means less time in the hospital. The cost of a doula is [$xxx.xx], while the cost of one day at [name of your local hospital] is [$xxx.xx].

I hired a doula to [put here your specific reasons, for example, to have a nonmedicated birth, to be able to stay on bed rest, to cope with postpartum depression, etc. Think in terms of what saves insurance companies money.]

And my doula achieved these goals. I avoided [narcotic or epidural medication, induction, c-section, etc.] as a result of my doula's support, saving your insurance company a significant amount of money.

I have included with my letter some papers on the research on doulas. Please take the time to read over them, and I'm sure you will see how doulas can help reduce costs for your company.

Sincerely,
[Your name here]

# Appendix 3
## Interview Guide for Hiring a Postpartum Doula

Feel free to photocopy this questionnaire to help interview potential doulas. The questions are only a guideline. You may have questions not listed below, or some questions here may not be relevant to your situation. For more detailed information on hiring a postpartum doula, see chapter 11.

## Phone Interview Guide

Name of Doula: _____

Phone number (_____)_____-_____

E-mail address: _____

Additional contact information: _____

_____

_____

If the doula says this is a bad time, schedule to call another time.

Date: _____  Time: _____

QUESTIONS TO ASK DURING PHONE INTERVIEW:

1. What kind of training and experience as a doula have you had?

_____

_____

_____

2. How would you define the postpartum doula's role?

_____

_____

_____

3. Please tell me about the services you offer.

_____

_____

_____

4. What do you charge for your services? Do you charge for a consultation meeting?

_____

_____

_____

5. Do you help with housework? Siblings? Run errands? Do you offer night care?

_____

_____

_____

6. Can you provide me with a couple names and phone numbers of previous clients, for references?

_____

_____

_____

ADDITIONAL QUESTIONS AND NOTES:

_____

_____

_____

_____

If you decide to meet with the doula in-person:

When: _____

Where you plan to meet with your doula: _____

Directions to the meeting place: _____

_____

_____

# Doula Interview Guide

Use this as a guide when you meet with any potential doulas. While part of your goal is to find out what services this doula offers, the most important part of the interview is to decide if her personality is a good fit. Do you feel comfortable with her? Do you like her?

Name of Doula: _____

Phone number (_____)_____-_____

E-mail address: _____

Additional contact information: _____

_____

When asking these questions, pay more attention to her way of speaking, her personality and her overall attitude, than to her specific answers.

- Why did you go into doula work?
- (If she is a mother herself) Can you tell me what you personally needed most after the birth of your child(ren)? Did you have any support?
- What is the most challenging aspect of your work as a doula?
- What do you see as your main role as my postpartum doula?
- How will you help my partner/family/older children?
- How can you help me deal with family problems or pushy guests?
- How do you feel about helping with practical needs, like dishes or cooking?

## DETAILS OF HER SERVICES:

Do you meet with me before the baby is born? If yes, what do you usually talk about with clients at this meeting? And is there a charge?

_____

_____

_____

At what point do you begin supporting me postpartum? How do I contact you?

_____

_____

_____

Can I expect you to be available during the two weeks before and after my expected due date? For how long can you act as my doula? How many hours per day, days per week, are you available? Any particular time of day?

_____

_____

_____

Do you have a back-up doula? If yes, under what circumstances do you call her? Can I meet with her? Can I have her contact information?

_____

_____

_____

What services do you offer? I need the most help with (_____). (Example: older children, housework, meals, night care, breast-feeding, etc.) How will you help with this?

_____

_____

_____

Do you offer any optional or extra services? (Ex. Night care services, run errands, etc.) How much do these extra services cost?

_____

_____

_____

What do you usually bring to help your clients? (For example, a baby sling or carrier, massages oils, etc.)

_____

_____

Do you help with breastfeeding? How?

_____

_____

_____

What are the terms of your contract? How do we schedule the days
and hours that you'll work? What are the payment terms?

_____

_____

_____

NOTES FOR ANY SPECIAL QUESTIONS YOU HAVE:
*(Tip: Write down any special questions here before you go to the*
*meeting.)*

_____

_____

_____

_____

_____

_____

_____

_____

# ——————Appendix 4——————
## Interview Guide for
## Hiring an Antepartum Doula

FEEL FREE TO PHOTOCOPY this questionnaire to help interview potential doulas. The questions are only a guideline. You may have questions not listed below, or some questions here may not be relevant to your situation. For more detailed information on hiring an antepartum doula, see chapter 12

## Phone Interview Guide

Name of Doula: _____

Phone number (_____)_____-_____

E-mail address: _____

Additional contact information: _____

_____

If the doula says this is a bad time, schedule to call another time.

Date: _____ Time: _____

QUESTIONS TO ASK DURING PHONE INTERVIEW:

1. What kind of training and experience as a doula have you had?

_____

_____

_____

2. Do you have any personal experience with bed rest/teen pregnancy/(whatever your concern is)? OR What do you think about teenage pregnancy?

_____

_____

_____

3. Please tell me about the services you offer. Do you offer labor doula services as well?

_____

_____

_____

4. What do you charge for your services?

_____

_____

_____

5. Do you help with housework? Siblings? Run errands? Will you help out at my home, while I'm in the hospital?

_____

_____

_____

6. Can you provide me with a couple names and phone numbers of previous clients, for references?

_____

_____

_____

ADDITIONAL QUESTIONS AND NOTES:

_____

_____

_____

_____

If you decide to meet with the doula in-person:

When: _____

Where you plan to meet with your doula: _____

Directions to the meeting place: _____

_____

_____

## Doula Interview Guide

Use this as a guide when you meet with any potential doulas. While part of your goal is to find out what services this doula offers, the most important part of the interview is to decide if her personality is a good fit. Do you feel comfortable with her? Do you like her?

Name of Doula: _____

Phone number (\_\_\_\_\_)\_\_\_\_\_-_____

E-mail address: _____

Additional contact information: _____

_____

When asking these questions, pay more attention to her way of speaking, her personality and her overall attitude, than to her specific answers.

- Why did you go into doula work?
- (If she has personally experienced your current situation before) Can you tell me about the most difficult part of bed rest/teen pregnancy/(your current problem) was for you? What birth memory do you cherish most?
- What is the most challenging aspect of your work as a doula?
- What do you see as your main role?
- How will you help my partner/family/older children?
- How do you feel about helping with practical needs, like dishes, cooking?

DETAILS OF HER SERVICES:

Do you offer phone support while you're working with me? When and how often can I call? Under what circumstances?

_____

_____

_____

How do I contact you? Can I expect you to be available during the two weeks before and after my expected due date?

_____

_____

_____

Do you have a back-up doula? If yes, under what circumstances do you call her? Can I meet with her? Can I have her contact information?

_____

_____

_____

What services do you offer? I need the most help with (_____). (Example: information on high risk pregnancy, emotional support, older children, housework, meals, night care, breastfeeding, etc.) How will you help with this?

_____

_____

_____

Do you offer any optional or extra services? (Photography, video, belly casting, night care, etc.) How much do these extra services cost, or are they included in the overall price?

_____

_____

_____

Do you offer labor support? How is this charged? (Consider asking questions from the labor doula interview guide, if you want your antepartum doula to provide labor support as well.)

_____

_____

_____

How long after the birth will you be available? Do you help with breastfeeding? What type of support do you provide postpartum? Can you help if I have a premature baby?

_____

_____

_____

What are the terms of your contract? How do we schedule the days and hours that you'll work? What are the payment terms?

_____

_____

_____

NOTES FOR ANY SPECIAL QUESTIONS YOU HAVE:
*(Tip: Write down any special questions here before you go to the meeting.)*

_____

_____

_____

_____

_____

_____

_____

# Appendix 5
## Organization Contact Information

NATIONAL DOULA ORGANIZATION WEB SITES AND
CONTACT INFORMATION

ALACE—The Association of Labor Assistants and Childbirth
Educators
P.O. Box 382724
Cambridge, MA 02238
(617) 441 - 2500
E-mail: alacehq@aol.com
www.alace.org

BBI—Birth and Bonding International
1126 Solano Ave.
Albany, CA 94706
(510) 527 - 2121
E-mail: bbint@flash.net
www.birthbonding.org

Birthing From Within
123 Wellesley SE
Albuquerque, NM 87106
(505) 254 - 4884
E-mail: contact@birthingfromwithin.com
www.birthpower.com

Birth Works
P.O. Box 2045
Medford, NJ 08055
(888) TO - BIRTH (862 - 4784)
E-mail: info@birthworks.org
www.birthworks.org

CAPPA—Childbirth and Postpartum Professional Association
PO Box 491448
Lawrenceville GA 30043
1-888-548-3672
E-mail: info@cappa.net
www.cappa.net

CEF—Childbirth Enhancement Foundation
1004 George Ave.
Rockledge, FL 32955
(321) 631 - 9977
E-mail: info@cefcares.org
www.cefcares.org

DONA—Doulas of North America
PO Box 626
Jasper, IN 47547
(801) 756 - 7331
E-mail: doula@dona.org
www.dona.org

ICEA—The International Childbirth Education Association
PO Box 20048
Minneapolis, Minnesota 55240
(952) 854 - 8660 or 1-800-827-ICEA
E-mail: info@icea.org
www.icea.org

National Association of Postpartum Care Services
800 Detroit St.
Denver, CO 80206
1-800-45-DOULA
E-mail: DoulaCare@aol.com
www.napcs.org

## CHILDBIRTH EDUCATION WEB SITES AND CONTACT INFORMATION

American Academy of Husband-Coached Childbirth (Bradley Method)
Box 5224
Sherman Oaks, CA 91413-5224
(800) 4-A-BIRTH or (818) 788-6662
www.bradleybirth.com

Birthing From Within
123 Wellesley SE
Albuquerque, NM 87106
(505) 254 - 4884
E-mail: contact@birthingfromwithin.com
www.birthpower.com

Birth Works
P.O. Box 2045
Medford, NJ 08055
(888) TO - BIRTH (862 - 4784)
E-mail: info@birthworks.org
www.birthworks.org

ICEA—The International Childbirth Education Association
PO Box 20048
Minneapolis, Minnesota 55240
(952) 854 - 8660 or 1-800-827-ICEA
E-mail: info@icea.org
www.icea.org

Lamaze International
2025 M Street, Suite 800
Washington DC 20036-3309
(202) 367-1128 or (800) 368-4404
E-mail: lamaze@dc.sba.com
www.lamaze-childbirth.com

## INTERNET LINKS

Because the Internet is always changing, links that are active now may be dead by the time this book is published. Please visit my web site at www.doyoudoula.com for a links to Web sites on pregnancy, birth, and postpartum topics.

# References

## Chapter 1

Campero, Lourdes, Cecilia Garcia, Carmen Diaz, Olivia Ortiz, Sofia Reynoso, & Ana Langer. "'Alone, I wouldn't have known what to do': A qualitative study on social support during labor and delivery in Mexico," *Social Science Medicine 47* (1998): 395–402.

Klaus, M. H., J. H. Kennell, and P. Klaus. *Mothering the Mother.* Cambridge, MA: Perseus Books, 1993: 3.

Springer, N. P., & C. V. Weel. Home birth: Safe in selected women, and with adequate infrastructure and support. Retrieved December 2, 2002 from World Wide Web, BMJ: http://bmj.com/archive/7068e.htm

## Chapter 2

Campero, Lourdes, Cecilia Garcia, Carmen Diaz, Olivia Ortiz, Sofia Reynoso, & Ana Langer. "Alone, I wouldn't have known what to do": A qualitative study on social support during labor and delivery in Mexico. *Social Science Medicine 47* (1998): 395–402.

Crowell, M., P. Hill, & S. Humenick. Relationship between obstetric analgesia and time of effective breast feeding, *Journal of Nurse Midwifery 39 no. 3* (1994): 150–6.

Eisenberg, A., H. E. Murkoff, & S. E. Hathaway. *What to Expect When You're Expecting.* New York: Workman Publishing Company, 1996: 228–29.

England, P., & Horowitz, R. *Birthing from Within.* New Mexico: Partera Press, 1998: 246–51.

Gordon, Nancy P., David Walton, Eileen McAdams, Judy Derman, Gina Gallitero, & Lynda Garrett. "Effects of providing hospital-based doulas in health maintenance organization hospitals." *Obstetrics & Gynecology 93, no. 3* (1999): 422–26.

Hodnett, E., & R. Osborn. Effects of continuous intrapartum professional support on childbirth outcomes. Research in Nursing and Health *12* (1989): 289–297.

Hofmeyr, G. J., V. C. Nikodem, W. Wolman, B. E. Chalmers, & T. Kramer. Companionship to modify the clinical birth environment: Effects on progress and perceptions of labour and breast-feeding. *British Journal of Obstetrics and Gynaecology 98* (1991): 756–764.

Jukelevics, N. A doula at your birth. Retrieved May 30, 2002, from the World Wide Web: http://www.vbac.com/doulaatyourbirth.html

Kennell J., M. Klaus, S. McGrath, S. Robertson, & C. Hinkley. Continuous emotional support during labor in a U.S. hospital: A randomized controlled trial. *Journal of the American Medical Association, 265* (1991): 2197–2201.

Menacker, F., & S. Curtin. Trends in cesarean birth and vaginal birth after previous cesarean, 1991–99. Retrived May 30, 2002 from World Wide Web, Center for Disease Control: http://www.cdc.gov/nchs/data/nvsr/nvsr49/nvsr49_13.pdf

Mortensen, E., K. Michaelsen, S. Sanders, & J. Reinisch. The association between duration of breastfeeding and adult intelligence. *Journal of the American Medical Association 287, No.18* (2002): 2365–71.

Ransjö-Arvidson, A., A. Matthiesen, G. Lilja, E. Nissen, A. Widström, & K. Uvnäs-Moberg. Maternal analgesia during labor disturbs newborn behavior: Effects on breastfeeding, temperature, and crying. *Birth 28, No. 1* (2001): 5–12.

Scott, K., G. Berkowitz, & M. Klaus. A comparison of intermittent and continuous support during labor: A meta-analysis. *Ameri-*

can *Journal of Obstetrics and Gynecology 180, No. 5*
(1999):1054–1059.

## Chapter 4

Klaus, M. H., & J. H. Kennell. The doula: An essential ingredient of childbirth rediscovered. *Acta Paediatrica 86* (1997): 1034–6.

## Chapter 12

Brown, D. *CAPPA Position Paper: Antepartum Doula Support for High-Risk Pregnancies.* Retrieved November 14, 2002, from the World Wide Web: www.childbirthprofessional.com/Docs/CAPD%20Position%20Paper%20pdf.pdf

# Acknowledgments

I WOULD LIKE TO acknowledge the following people:

- The editors and designers at Prima Publishing. Specifically, Jamie Miller, who approached me with the idea for this book and allowed me to take on the project, and Andi Reese Brady, my project editor, who helped make this book great and always patiently and timely answered my questions.
- My photographers, Stephanie Soderblom and Marilyn Nolt, for coming through, even at the last minute, and taking great photos. Thank you to tracy hartley from BestDoulas.com, who provided a few photos, and to Lucky Tomaszek, who allowed me to publish a photo from her homebirth.
- Polly Perez, an amazing author, speaker, nurse, and doula, for taking the time to read and review the book.
- Mayer Eisenstein, M.D., for agreeing to write the foreword.
- Sharon Quarrington and Georganne Hampton, for sharing their birth stories and allowing me to publish them in the book.
- My writing friends on Momwriters.com. I wouldn't be where I am today without you. Specifically, thank you my writing partner, Phyllis Ring, who inspired me in so many ways and did a wonderful job of editing many of my chapters. Thank you to Lisa Beamer, for motivating me and pushing me to meet my goals. Thank you also to Shae, Teri, Rebecca, Heather, Michelle, Kristen, Kelly, Kathleen, Dena, and Apryl,

Momwriters who took the time to read through and comment on my work.

- My co-workers at Myria Media, Inc., and ePregnancy Magazine. Nancy Price, Betsy Gartrell-Judd and Jennifer Newton Reents, for your amazing patience! And for your priceless help with publicity through ePregnancy Magazine.
- Sara Kanant, for letting me talk through writer's block, inspiring me, and babysitting my son when I feel asleep from a late night of work. (We miss you!)
- My daddy, who carefully read each chapter, making suggestions and corrections. And my mommy, who bragged about me and my book to all her friends, selling a few copies before the book was even published!
- My husband, for taking the kids on outings so I could write, for not complaining too much when I had to stay up late "again," for putting up with simple dinners and hiring a maid, for reading through my work and making corrections, for praying for me, and . . . well, there are not enough words to describe how much I owe you! And my children, for always providing inspiration.
- My doula, Diane Lentine. Thank you showing me how great a doula-supported birth can be.
- All the moms, doulas, nurses, doctors, and childbirth professionals who took time from their busy days to answer my never-ending list of questions. Specifically, thank you to Amy Adams, Jennifer Adkins, Donna Algiere, Shereen Allen, Tony Allen, Carrie Asuncion, Julie Baker, Connie Banack, Patricia Battle, Karen Beiley, Kimberly Bepler, Anna Berger, Kathryn Berkowitz, Rose Marie Bertrand, Kris Evans Bien, Jamie R. Blake, Christa Marie Bobrowski, Michelle Handschuh Bork, Melanie Bowden, Kate Brett, Rachel Brown, Ruth Bryskier, Adam Burch, Melanie Burch, Ann Marie K. Burkhart, Kari Butcher, Teri Castillo, Jessie Catacutan,

Kimberlee Catacutan, Alissa Catalan, Eileen Chevalier, Kathy
M. Clark, Mary Kathryn Clark, Angie Claussen, Sue Coffman,
Anna Colpitts, Susan Cooper, Barbara A. Coscia, Michelle
Handschuh Cousins, Susanne Cousins, Mary Craig, Ken
Crounse, Jane Cruice, ParisAnne Dallet, Nick Dallett, Laura
Dana, Karen Davis, Wendy Newhouse Davis, Jennifer
DeLugach, Frank J. DeMarco, Michael Dickson, Anita Don-
aldson, Sarah Ebert, Suzanne Evans, DeeDee Farris-Folkerts,
Dina LeAnn Fischer, Krishna Fogle, Susan Fraga, Chana B.
Frydman, Sarah C. de la Fuente, Ann Fuller, Rebecca Gal-
lagher, Kathy Galt, Mark Galt, Dr. Greg Gelburd, Mireille
Ghercioiu, Trish Gibson-Grossmann, Alice Gilgoff, Jessica
Gill, Dan Glassman, Peri Goldberg, Andrea Golden, Koren
Gould, Kimberly Govekar, Rosanne Gregory, Claire Grop-
man, Marlene Gubler, Denise Gustafson, Amy Guzules,
Charlene Hamilton-Biggs, Robin Harris, Tracy Hartley, Lori
Harvey, Monte Harvey, Jesse Remer Henderson, Dan Herrick,
Staci Herrick, Anne Hicks, Byron Hicks, Yolonda Washing-
ton High, Ana Hill, Annemarie La Vie Hodges, Dara Hogue,
Don Hogue, Susan Michele Hollis-Dickson, Amy Holsinger,
Tiffany Hoopert, Barbara A. Hotelling, Teresa Howard, Mark
Howell, Traci Howell, Harmony Hutman, Seairth Jacobs,
Dianne Kasten, Mark Kasten, Lauren L. Keim, Kelli Keough,
Marilee Kinsella, Heather M. Kleber, Laura Knittel, Cathy
Koos, Brenda Kotecki-Rocklin, Debbie Kozell, Sarah
Krauskopf, Bianca Kurti, Judy Lage, Lori Laken, Jennifer
Larrabee, Debbie Lavin, Virginia L'Bassi, Yonit Lea, Renata
Lebbe, Lori Lee, Dianne Lentine, Steve Levin, Bonnie L.
Liegey, Paula Lilly, Connie Livingston, Billy Long, Rachel
Long, Elizabeth Lott, Colleen Saint Loup, Lorraine Lucas,
Jeanette Lundgren, Miriam Martin, Uta Mattox, Christi
Maybray, Elspeth McClanahan, Kim McGuire, Jean
McHenry, Jennifer McQuillan, LaNette J. McQuitty, Wendy

A. Middleton, Melanie R. Miner, Michelle Minnich, Steve Minnich, Valerie Moore, Sandra Mort, Christine Morton, David Moskowitz, Katrin Moskowitz, Stephanie Mulfinger, Emily Murray, Monica Murray, Jessica Naditch, Andre L. Narbonne, Julie Elizabeth Baker Nolan, Hillary Noyes-Keene, Kelley O'Briant, Paula Oakes, Heather Ockert, Jennifer E.B. Ogburn, Sue Opahle, Erin Pavlina, Lauralynn Pearson, Jennifer Pells, Amy Pepe, Leonard Pepe, Polly Perez, Jennifer Pettit, Shirley M. Picard, Terri Plewa, Dwight Polglaze, Julie Polglaze, Melody Possinger, Jennifer Powers, Jennifer S. Powers, Lynn Prepejchal, Lori Ratchin, Shurene Rehmke, Michael Reno, Sara Roberts, Lynn Rosser, Darlene Rowe, Hank Rowe, Elizabeth A. D. Rutherfurd, Crystal Sada, Elaine Sargent, Martha Scheer, Karen Schroeder, Andrea Schumann, Jill Scobie, Jerrod Sessler, Nikki Sessler, Jodi Baker Shair, Leslie Shapiro, Devorah Shulman, Rachel Silber, Penny Simkin, Marc Sinclair, Ben Smallwood, Emily Smallwood, DeeDee Smith, Kira Smith, Lisa Sommer, Julia Spencer, Wendy Spry, Shannon Stainer, Ilana Stein, Esther Stroh, Megan Tarnow, Kim Thomas, Karen Thorpe, Lucky Tomaszek, Tabitha Trotter, Kathy Urban, Tina Vanasse, Carrie VanDuzee, William A. VanDuzee, Kerry Vaughan, Jen Velazquez, Sarah Wayland, Leslie Webb, Ashley Wedgman, Curt White, Jennifer White, Liza White, Cyndi Whitwell, Jennifer Wisenbaker, Kimberly Wright, Elizabeth Wyatt, Mary Wyman, Vicky York, Ina, and "Suaad Ali's dad."

- Most important, I acknowledge G-d. Without His help, none of this could have happened. And only with His help will this book go on to to help others.

# Index